SANDRA L. VASHER

I Hear Some People Just Have Sex

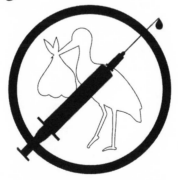

AN INFERTILITY MEMOIR
WITH AN AMBIGUOUS ENDING

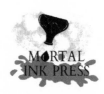

MORTAL
INK PRESS

I HEAR SOME PEOPLE JUST HAVE SEX

For information, please contact Mortal Ink Press LLC, PO Box 30811, Raleigh, NC 27622-0811, USA.

www.mortalinkpress.com

ISBN 978-1-950989-11-9 (paperback)

ISBN 978-1-950989-12-6 (ebook)

ISBN 978-1-950989-13-3 (audiobook)

This book is dedicated to the babies we lost.
Your lives were precious to us. Your souls are not forgotten.

TABLE OF CONTENTS

Infertility Changes Everything

The Really Hard Parts

Someone Has It Worse

Expect the Unexpected...

Useful Info

FOREWORD
By John-Malcolm M. Cox

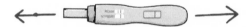

I'm writing this from the back deck on a gorgeous 70-degree late-November Carolina Saturday. Football is on the TV, and perhaps fittingly for these strange times, Indiana is somehow ranked No. 9 and giving Ohio State a run for its money. Just when you thought 2020 couldn't get weirder. But here I am because Sandy has been nagging me for several weeks[1] to write a foreword for her book. I've been procrastinating, and apparently, the "deadline" is now tomorrow.[2]

I've been procrastinating because I have no idea what to say. How does one write a foreword to a book about infertility? Put differently, how does a man write a forward to his wife's memoir about infertility? I honestly have no idea.

I'm a child of the 1980s, raised by parents who were born during the Second World War and came of age when America still did great things. Above all, my parents instilled in me a strong, forward-looking work ethic. "Put your hand to the plow and don't look back," my mother would say.[3]

---

1   (More like months. ~Sandy)
2   (He was granted many extensions.)
3   Like many colloquial sayings, this phrase has its roots in the

And thank goodness she did. As a result, I'm not a millennial weenie with an overabundance of "feelings" constantly bubbling up due to things that happened in the past. I don't do feelings, or at least not feelings that I wear on my sleeve.

What I do instead is thoughts. So here are some thoughts—three, actually, and in reverse order of importance—about our infertility journey.

Infertility is about the meaning of life. A few years ago, right while we were in the middle of infertility hell, there was a commercial for an insurance company that seemed to run whenever I turned on the TV. It started with a guy in his mid-20s, at a party, checking out a hot girl. He turns to his buddies and says, "I'm never getting married."

Predictably, the commercial then cuts to him buying a ring for his soon-to-be wife and progresses through various other juxtapositions ("We're never having kids"/cut to wife in labor; "We're never moving to the suburbs"/cut to him doing yard work; etc.) until it ends with him in his late-30s sitting on a couch with his wife, two kids asleep on his lap, and a minivan in his driveway. He says, "I'm never letting go." Despite its previous juxtapositions, I suppose the commercial intends to convey that he has found the meaning of his life and is content.[4]

Bible. *See* Luke 9:62 New Revised Standard Version ("Jesus said to him, 'No one who puts a hand to the plow and looks back is fit for the kingdom of God.'"). But for my mother, a first-generation American whose Scotch parents and grandparents broke the Canadian plains, the phrase was applied as aptly to industry as to faith.

4   That being said, because the commercial also implies he sold a 1967 Camaro SS to buy his minivan, it could be this dude is about to have a major mid-life crisis. If commercials had alternate endings, this one would cut to him blasting across

I can relate to a portion of this commercial. As a mid-20s bachelor living and working in downtown Chicago, I spent many weekends with my friends, living it up, stumbling home to my condo, and doing it all again the next week. Predictably, life progressed to meeting and marrying Sandy and moving out of the city to a house in suburban Atlanta. But for us, that is where the commercial paused. Sandy was never in labor. There were never any kids asleep on my lap.[5]

Of course, what this means is that there was also no "I'm never letting go." But that is okay. Over the last decade, we have found meaning and contentment in other ways. Throughout this book, you will read about some of our many adventures and hobbies and how infertility has provided the opportunity to find meaning in more than just kids.

Infertility is about courage. There is, however, a reason why a chief marketing officer at an insurance company decided to spend millions of dollars to run that commercial *a• nauseum* during a whole host of sporting events watched primarily by men in their 30s and 40s. Having kids, and finding meaning and contentment in them, is normal. It is so normal, in fact, that one of my old friends from Chicago recently told me that having kids is "the" meaning of life. He now has three.[6]

What is scary for someone facing infertility is that my friend might be right. Despite the meaning we have found, as I have gotten older, I worry about what the future holds.

---

the Southwest desert in a Corvette convertible with the hot girl from the party in the passenger seat.

5   I guess the good news is that I didn't sell our British sports cars to buy a minivan.

6   None of this is meant to be critical, so please don't read it that way. I love my friend like a brother and could not be happier for him and his wife.

Will our hobbies and adventures give us fulfillment as we grow old? What will we think about when we are dying? Will anyone be there? Will anyone care? Will we be forgotten? What legacy will we leave for the world?

Infertility is about facing these fears. It is about having the courage to admit that you actually, and desperately, want the normal. It is about having the courage to go for it despite the odds. It is about going to appointments, talking to doctors, holding your wife's hand during procedures, and waiting for news, all while knowing you may never get that perfect family cuddled up on the couch. And perhaps more than anything, it is about being courageous in the face of bad news, putting your hand to the plow and moving forward with the life you have built instead of looking back to what might have been.

Infertility is about love. After leaving the altar at our wedding, I turned to Sandy and said, "This is the best decision I ever made." Within two years, we were on the verge of divorce. But we persevered, and I now cannot imagine my life without her. My love for her grows every day, in part because of our infertility journey.

I'm incredibly lucky to have a loving and caring wife who has been willing to go through so much just so we could try to have a family with kids together. Even more than that, I'm lucky to have someone who has the courage to face fears and have faith that, even without kids, we can find meaning and contentment together.

I hope you enjoy her story. I hope it makes you laugh, cry, and provides some insight into how at least one couple has managed through nearly a decade of bad news and loss. I also hope that it helps you find meaning, courage, and love in your journey. Infertility is not a tragedy. It is just a part of life for some couples. Although we don't yet know how our journey ends, what I do know is that despite the loss and hardship we have faced, I would not trade the meaning, courage, and, most importantly, love for Sandy that I have found along the way. Happy reading.

John-Malcolm M. Cox
The husband.

PART I

Infertility 101

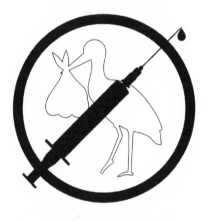

We want far better reasons for having children than not knowing how to prevent them.
~ Dora Winifred Black Russell

CHAPTER ONE
This is Me. In a Storm

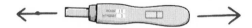

A TYPICAL VISIT TO A FERTILITY CLINIC

It's the indignity of it all. That's what I think. That's what I'm thinking as a doctor moves my knees apart, warns me that I'm going to feel a push, and inserts a probe that's a lot bigger than any sex toy I've ever owned up my vagina.

It doesn't hurt. This is far from being my first pelvic ultrasound, and I know the drill cold, start to finish.

You show up at your fertility clinic, check in, sit down, and don't make eye contact with any of the other women or couples waiting there. There are always at least four other people, often more, because the clinic moves patients in and out all day long. Someone brought a baby in today because apparently, she has no sense of decency. Or possibly she has no childcare, but you're not in the mood to feel sympathetic. This is a fertility clinic. It is the last place where you want to watch other women hold or play with the happy babies they were able to deliver.

Thankfully, this isn't like an obstetrician-gynecologist (ob/gyn) appointment where you have to wait forever for your turn. You barely have time to glower once at the woman with the baby and check your email before a nurse calls your name.

"Sandra Vasher?" she says. The nurse looks young, and she's carrying a clipboard. You get up and follow her back into the clinic. She confirms your birthday while you walk and leads you into a small, dark room with a raised examination table, an ultrasound machine, and a connected bathroom.

"Empty your bladder, undress from the waist down, sheet goes over your lap, the doctor will be here in a minute," the nurse says, barely looking at you while you set down your purse on the stool they put near the top edge of the exam table. That stool is for your partner to sit in, but if your husband came to all these appointments with you, he would no longer have a job. This is a routine appointment, so you are, as usual, alone.

You go to the bathroom, pee fast, wash your hands, and check to make sure you didn't accidentally leave any toilet paper behind. Clarification: you check to make sure you didn't accidentally leave any toilet paper in your vagina. That's pretty much all you worry about leaving up there these days. It's been a while since you cared about whatever else the doctor might find. The doctors in these offices see blood, mucus, semen, and all sorts of pubic hairstyles. It doesn't really matter if you've shaved all your hair off, trimmed it neatly, or decided to go au naturel. It doesn't matter if you have piercings or tattoos. The medical professionals at a fertility clinic see dozens of vaginas every morning. You can rest assured that you don't have a special snowflake vagina.

Now that you've stripped everything from the waist

down off (except your socks—you keep those on because for God's sake, your socks are the last shred of physical dignity you're holding on to), you sit down on the puppy potty pad they put at the bottom edge of the examination table, pull the inadequate paper sheet over your thighs, and try not to slouch too much while you wait for the doctor.

He comes in. Or she. You don't have the same doctor each time. There are six in this office, and they take turns with these basic monitoring appointments.

The doctor says hello. Initially, you weren't sure if you should shake the doctor's hand or something as they enter the exam room. Your husband does that sometimes. But that seems weird for you, so you settle for trying not to look tense. This, after all, is something you are an old hat at. You are not stressed.

I repeat. You are not stressed.

You appreciate that the doctor puts a hefty amount of lube on that wand he's about to stick up inside you, and you consciously try to relax all the muscles in your pelvic region while the wand slides in. Trust me, it won't help anything if you clam up.

That's where I am now. Thinking about how much privacy I've lost thanks to infertility, right while a doctor maneuvers an uncomfortably long wand in my body and shows me a picture of my empty uterus.

He measures the lining of my uterus. I've been on birth control for several weeks, so it's as thin as they're expecting. The doctor jabs the wand left. Left ovary looks good. Jabs the wand right. Right ovary looks good.

The door opens. It's a nurse who has some questions for the doctor about your chart. There's another nurse in there with the doctor already, and the nurses rotate even more than the doctors, so I recognize one but not the other. It doesn't make a difference whether I have ever met them before. No matter how you slice it, three people I barely know still looked at my vagina today.

Don't even *try* to tell me that this is the same when you're pregnant. Pregnancy is limited to less than a year, and most of those ultrasounds are not transvaginal. Everyone gets a good look at your belly over and over, not your vagina. I will concede that labor and delivery involve plenty of people seeing things you probably never wanted anyone to see, but that happens once and with a lot of adrenalin and possibly an epidural. These factors are not present at a transvaginal ultrasound, and infertility can go on for years. I have had far more strangers look at my vagina than the young woman down the street who just had her first baby.

Since there is nothing spectacular about my ovaries or uterus today, the doctor pulls the wand out and tells me everything looks good. I'm left to put my pants back on, grab my checkout sheet, and head over to the lab for bloodwork. Over the course of a single frozen embryo in vitro fertilization (IVF) cycle, I will probably go through at least three appointments just like this. Usually, bloodwork to test my estrogen and/or progesterone levels comes along with the checks. I am a pin cushion during these cycles, and I have big veins, but I worry about whether having a needle stuck into the same vein so often might cause permanent damage.

The poor woman next to me looks like she's almost in tears. They're having trouble finding her vein. This reminds me that it is important for a woman going through this never to tell herself or anyone else that what she is going through is as bad as it can get. In the world of infertility, I can guarantee you, someone always has it worse.

I give the lab my blood, give that poor woman a sympathy glance, get up from the chair, and go check out. My health insurance doesn't cover most of this, so my husband and I had to pay upfront for the vast majority of this infertility cycle.

In total, with drugs and monitoring appointments and the embryo transfer itself and the pregnancy test at the end, this will run us about four-thousand dollars, which we consider cheap. If we had needed an egg retrieval first, we would have been in for more like twenty-thousand dollars.

Infertility is expensive.

Somehow, even though I pre-paid for this cycle, I still owe a thirty-dollar co-pay today, and I don't question any of this anymore. The fertility clinic is always right when it comes to how much money you owe them. I hand over my credit card—my personal credit card; we blew through the FSA card much earlier in the year with a million diagnostic tests—and I genuinely appreciate that the receptionist here always smiles and says gently, "Now you have a nice day."

"You, too," I tell her. I mean that. I like her.

I head to the parking lot, get in my car, text my husband to tell him everything was fine, and move on to the rest of my day. The whole appointment took twenty minutes. In and out just like that, though by the time I'm out I always feel somewhat dazed. I think because it's all just kind of surreal and again because of that lack of dignity. You disassociate a little while you're spread out like a chicken about to be roasted on an examination table. You try not to wince while they take blood again, you try not to think while you pay your bill. You try to snap out of that dissociative state as soon as possible when it is over because you don't want to go through life not feeling anything.

That's how I get through it. By trying to find the balance between feeling everything and feeling nothing. That is how I've done this for nearly a decade. By the time I wrote this memoir, I'd survived 16 infertility cycles.

That number includes four timed intercourse cycles, some with fertility drugs and some without anything but monitoring, and two intrauterine insemination (IUI) cycles with fertility drugs. It includes one fresh IVF cycle with egg retrieval followed by one fresh and three frozen embryo transfer cycles, plus a second fresh IVF cycle with egg retrieval followed by three frozen embryo transfer cycles. It includes two mock embryo transfer cycles.

I've had two miscarriages. I've had three pregnancies. I've never had a live birth, but I'm in an IVF cycle right now, as I write this story, and this is my third pregnancy, so this might be the one that makes it.

I'm thirty-nine years old, I started my infertility journey when I was thirty, and I do not yet have a baby in my arms.

If you're reading this book, I'm guessing it's because you're suffering through some of what I've gone through. Maybe you're going through infertility treatments yourself. Maybe your partner is going through the treatments, and you're suffering right alongside her.

Or if you're not the one trying to get pregnant, maybe you have a loved one—a daughter, a niece, a best friend, a cousin—going through this. Maybe you're afraid you're going to have to face something like this someday, and you want to know what you're up against. Maybe you are curious what all the fuss is about infertility. Maybe you just want someone to explain what the heck "IUI" and "IVF" even mean.

But probably you picked up this book because the nightmare that is infertility is affecting you personally. And if that is the case, I'm sorry you're here. Really, terribly sorry. Infertility is awful, and no matter how you're facing it, you're in for a bumpy ride. I hope for your sake that it is a short ride. If you're in it for the long haul, though, you came to the right place. I've had a long journey myself, and I have a lot of information to share.

This is my story, and I'll walk you through the whole thing in this book. My story has a lot of twists and turns to keep track of, and I hope it makes you laugh more than it makes you cry. I've tried to clearly explain the lingo of infertility as I go through these chapters, but if you get lost with the terminology, I recommend checking out the glossary in Appendix A at the back of the book. You can also read a condensed version of my entire chronology of infertility treatments, including how much time and money it all took, in Appendix B.

To clarify before we begin, this is not a "how to survive infertility and make it out on the other side" book. Those are written by people who've made it out. I am not one of those people. It is late 2020, and my husband and I started "trying" in 2012. I've gone through so many drugs and so many treatments. I've had multiple miscarriages, multiple egg retrievals, multiple in vitro fertilization cycles. I've been through the wringer.

I'm not done, either. I'm currently eight months pregnant, and you would think that would be long enough to rest easy, but it isn't. I've had too much go wrong before. My current pregnancy is too high-risk.

Even if this pregnancy results in a live birth—and I pray that it does—I still have one embryo frozen on ice. I do not know what will happen from here. If I have a baby in a few weeks, will I push forward with infertility treatments one day for a second baby? What if I do not have a baby? Will I try one last IVF cycle? Move on to adoption? Decide to live without children? I don't have those answers.

In other words: I can't tell you how to "get out" on the other side because I've never gotten out. I definitely can't give you a miracle cure that will guarantee you a baby. Nor can I teach you how to survive *until* you have a baby. I only know how to survive *while trying* to have a baby, and without any guarantees. Unfortunately, no one can guarantee anyone a baby. Babies are miracles, and you may never be blessed with that miracle. You may never get out on the other side. I may never get there.

But I'm in the same storm you are, and I'm sharing my story because I've been in this damned boat for long enough to know how not to sink. If you are reading this, I want you to know you can survive, too. Even if you have to stay here forever. You can learn how to steer this thing in a hurricane. You can learn how to see through your own tears. You can learn how to hang on when the worst waves threaten to rise over you and how to come back up for air if you go under.

I promise, you were made strong enough for this. You may be barren, but you are not broken. And I hope that you'll stick with me long enough to see that it goes beyond that.

Infertility is not a blessing. It is, however, something that will change you, and other than just being here with you as you fight hell and high water, I'm here because I want you to see that what you're going through has the potential to change you for the better.

I don't know when this is going to end for you. I know infertility will make you feel like you're drowning sometimes.

And then I know that there will be a day when you wake up with the realization that this has made you the kind of person who can get through *so much more* than you ever thought. I will not sugar coat anything for you here. I'm going to give you a real look at infertility. But I will also give you a real look at how you can survive and maybe even thrive in the midst of infertility treatments.

So now, let me show you how I've spent nearly all of the last decade hitching up my pants and removing them in front of everyone. This gets worse before it gets better, but if my story helps you, even just to feel less alone, then I am glad I shared it with you.

I hear some people just have sex to get pregnant.

Not me.

This is what I know about *not* being able to make babies, after eight and a half years of infertility.

CHAPTER TWO
The Sun, Moon & Stars

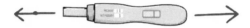

WISDOM I REJECTED

It is fall 2012, I'm thirty years old, I've been married for almost a year, and I'm sitting in my gynecologist's office. I have been nervous about this appointment for weeks. So nervous that I asked my husband, who is a lawyer, to help me prepare for it. I am also technically a lawyer, but he is far better than me when it comes to something like preparing for a trial, and that is what this feels like.

For the conversation I am about to have with my gynecologist, Malcolm gave me talking points, and we practiced until I could remember not to ramble or lose the plot. He says this is how he preps witnesses for trials, and I feel as prepared as I can be. I am still terrified.

This conversation should not be difficult. I have spent my entire life explaining to doctors that I *on't get perio*s. I have known for years that it could be difficult for me to have children. I *think* I have polycystic ovarian syndrome (PCOS), though technically, I've never been diagnosed. What the doctors write on my charts is just "amenorrhea." That means "no periods." No doctor has ever assigned a specific cause to that problem. They just prescribe birth control, and that fixes that. Then sometimes they say, "when you want to get pregnant, you'll probably need help." No doctor has ever explained exactly what help I need or exactly why I need help to begin with.

Now I want to get pregnant, but I'm not ready to start infertility treatments or anything extreme. First, I want to see if I can get my periods to start so that I can get pregnant the natural way. I've read that there's this drug, metformin, that can sometimes help women with PCOS. I asked my gynecologist about it in the spring at my annual appointment, but she told me metformin was unlikely to do anything to help me and that it would be better just to stay on birth control.

I was too afraid to fight my doctor in the spring. I don't know what it is about ob/gyns that scares me. Maybe I have some white coat syndrome. Maybe the fact that I had to start going to an ob/gyn when I was fifteen has something to do with it. Maybe it's that these doctors have so much power over my body in such an intimate way.

Whatever the case, it was a problem for me at my appointment in the spring. I walked away without the metformin and went off birth control without my doctor's help. Then my husband and I stopped using condoms and sort of hoped something would happen.

Of course, nothing happened. My periods never started. I bought that book, *Taking Charge of Your Fertility* by Toni Weschler, and I started tracking my basal body temperature, but my temperatures never changed enough to show I was ovulating. As far as I know, I don't ovulate and I don't have periods.

I made this appointment specifically to advocate for the metformin. I've done a ton of research. I've spoken with other doctors who are not ob/gyns. Metformin is a cheap drug that has some good side benefits and downsides that seem minimal to me. It is possible that it can restore my periods because sometimes it does that for women with PCOS. All I have to do is have this conversation where I persuade my doctor to let me try it.

Sweat drips from my armpits as I wait for the appointment to begin. I'm a sweaty, sweaty person. Excessively sweaty. As in, I can't wear just one t-shirt, even in the winter, or everyone will see my pit stains. I also have random hair on my chin that I have to pluck away, and I am always on a diet because I am never thin. These things—the sweating, the unwanted hair, the fat girl problems—are all symptoms of PCOS. Along with my total lack of periods, it seems like a pretty clear case to me.

If I am right that I have PCOS, I am exactly the person who should be trying metformin. I *know* I am. I have the Internet to back me up. And I believe that once my doctor prescribes the metformin, I will start taking it, and everything will change. A few months from now, I will be getting regular periods. Then, my husband and I can do what other couples do when they think they're ready for kids but don't want to go crazy yet. We can have sex whenever we want without using any protection and hope we get pregnant the old-fashioned way.

That would be wonderful. I already feel behind. In my ideal world, I was married at age twenty-seven and pregnant by now. I want four kids, spaced two-to-three years apart, and it would be best if I start now so that I have enough energy for all those kids.

I explain as much of this as I can to my gyno while I squeeze my arms to my sides and try not to look as sweaty and nervous as I actually am. She warns me again that metformin probably won't make my periods start. She says the dose I would need to make that happen could have unpleasant gastrointestinal side effects.

I ask her for the drug anyway, and I must sound either desperate or persuasive because she prescribes it. However, she ends the conversation by telling me one of the cruelest things a doctor has ever said to me. "You don't get to decide if you have children. No one does."

I walk out feeling crushed even though I have the prescription I came in for, and it's all I can do not to cry over what the doctor said. I rationalize it for the next few days. She's not telling me I *won't* have kids, right? She's telling me I need to set my expectations lower. Maybe I can't plan four children spaced out perfectly over eight years. Maybe I can't decide that I'll have two boys and two girls. I'll have kids, of course, but that kind of precision … I need to get over that.

I "adjust" my expectations. I start taking metformin. I never experience those gastrointestinal problems the doctor talked about, but I do eat slightly less on metformin for a few months. Half a year passes. I continue tracking my basal body temperature, taking the metformin, trying various diets to restore my periods. But I never ovulate, and my periods never come.

In spring of 2013, I return to my ob/gyn for my annual appointment. By now, I feel discouraged. Not being on birth control *oes* have negative side effects for me. Like more chin hair, less hair on the top of my head, and bad acne. I have awful, cystic acne scars all over my face, and all that acne happened in my late twenties. Now I'm over thirty, and I'm getting the same acne again. It's affecting my self-esteem.

Also, since the metformin didn't work, I now know that I need to see a fertility specialist if I want to get pregnant. Not right this second, though. Right this second, my husband and I are moving from our apartment in Chicago, Illinois, to a new home in Marietta, Georgia. In the meanwhile, I want back on birth control. Clearly, we're not getting pregnant, and I'm tired of the bad side effects that birth control can fix. Anyway, I have plenty of time for babies. A fertility specialist can help me after we get to Georgia.

My ob/gyn grins when I ask her to put me back on birth control. She says, "You want back on the good stuff, huh?" and she has no problem prescribing both the birth control and the metformin this time, since I'm not experiencing negative side effects from the metformin but I am losing some weight. That is the last time I see that doctor. It will be years before I understand how wise she was.

A FREQUENTLY ASKED QUESTION

I'm worried I may have trouble getting pregnant. What can I do to make sure I'm able to have babies?

ANSWER: FIND A DOCTOR YOU TRUST

There's more to that answer, obviously, but before I get into that—and before I get much further into this book—let's start with something pretty basic that you need to know.

I'm not a doctor, and neither is my husband.

If you missed it above, we're lawyers. Or he's a lawyer, and I'm an ex-lawyer-turned-writer-and-serial-entrepreneur.

One of the biggest problems with infertility as a societal issue is that there is no one-size-fits-all treatment, and yet, as soon as you embark on this journey, you are likely to get a plethora of unwanted advice about how to treat your infertility. The advice will come from all kinds of non-experts who assume you both need and want their opinion about how you can get pregnant.

The vast majority of the advice will be bad. In many cases, it won't even come from someone who's struggled with infertility! As if a woman (or a man) who has never had to work to get pregnant (or get someone pregnant) knows anything about what actually made that miracle happen!

Worse, while some of this bad advice will come from random acquaintances who barely know anything about you except that you are a "certain age" and you do not yet have children, some advice will come from people you love and trust. Your mother, your grandmother, your sister, your cousin, your best friend, your old college roommate. You will want to listen to them. Their voices will stick in your head. But they will only sometimes know anything about what is causing your infertility problems or how you should treat those problems.

Here is some sage wisdom: when it comes to how your body works, what medical problems you might have that could prevent you from getting pregnant, what treatments might help you get pregnant, or really *anything* related to infertility and your specific body, you cannot rely on anyone who is not your doctor to give you good advice.

Your neighbor's best friend's sister who lives in Ohio and

has a cousin who has a yoga instructor who knows a woman who tried to get pregnant for years and then went to a clinic in Canada where they told her exactly what *you* should do to get pregnant is not a trustworthy source of information.

Seriously.

Start learning right this second to plug your ears and sing "la la la" every time some kind person who is just *so heartbroken* by your barren despair tries to give you advice about your infertility as if they are an expert when they don't even know what you have already discussed with your doctor.

Try to forgive these people. They mean well, and if you can't forgive them, you'll probably be angry at half the world before this is over. Forgiveness is good for you.

But the point is, if you're having trouble getting pregnant, the last thing you need is for some ill-informed, self-proclaimed "expert" to give you medical advice about your infertility problems. The only medical advice you should be taking about your reproductive system is the advice your doctors give you. Your doctor is a professional. Your doctor is the one you need to trust. If you do not trust your doctor, you need a second opinion.

And P.S., when I say "doctor" here, I'm talking about your reproductive endocrinologist, not your ob/gyn or your family doctor. Your normal doctors might be amazing, but they don't have nearly the training a reproductive endocrinologist has about infertility, and they can inadvertently lead you astray because of this.

Google is not your doctor. Your mom is (probably) not your doctor. And, very importantly, I am not your doctor. Please do not take this book as a tool you can use to diagnose yourself. The advice I have is not advice that will help you get pregnant. It is advice that will help you withstand your own infertility journey. It is about coping, not treating. Big difference there.

Now, for my first tangible piece of coping advice ...

INFERTILITY LESSON #1

If you think you might have trouble getting pregnant, find a local fertility clinic and set up a consult with a reproductive endocrinologist. Now.

Do not wait years to get help.

The American Society for Reproductive Medicine (ASRM) says couples should usually seek medical help if they cannot get pregnant after a year of unprotected sex. But if you are over the age of thirty-five and you have been trying for six months, that's long enough, and if you have some reason to think you might not be able to get pregnant—like you don't get periods—then you should get help immediately.[1]

In case this lesson isn't abundantly clear: do not wait. As you will see in later chapters of this book or as soon as you see a reproductive endocrinologist for the first time, infertility is the longest waiting game you'll ever play. You don't need to make it worse by adding a delay at the beginning of the game. Anyway, it is far better to know early what you're dealing with than to wait and discover too late that you're, you know, *too late.*

Caution: a good reproductive endocrinologist isn't likely to have immediate availability. It can take *weeks* to get an initial consultation with a good doctor, especially in a busy area. If you're worried about getting pregnant, start researching reproductive endocrinologists and fertility clinics in your area. Put this on your to-do list for this week. Or hell, set down this book, do your research, call that clinic today, and ask to set up an initial consultation.

Need help finding a reproductive endocrinologist? The American Society for Reproductive Medicine has a website with a lot of great information and resources and also a "find a health professional" tab. Here is the website: https://www. reproductivefacts.org/.

HOW BABIES ARE MADE

Now, even though I just told you to find a doctor you can trust to give you information about what you personally need to do to make babies, I know you're still going to do a lot of Googling if you're worried about this. Even if you don't employ the power of the Internet in a desperate attempt to learn how to get pregnant when you can't, you'll get lots of advice about how to do it from people who know little more than what they learned in middle school sex-ed about how to make babies.

In case you didn't know, sex-ed in America is atrocious at best and totally absent at worst.[2]

So let me be presumptuous for a minute and assume you're somewhere near the beginning of your infertility journey. You want to know what you must do to get pregnant, right? Or you want to know what you're doing wrong that you're not getting pregnant. You want diagrams, charts, research, maybe a Magic 8-Ball, anything that will give you some concrete, yes or no answers about what exactly you need to do if you want a baby a year from now.

Okay, well, without giving you a diagnosis, there is something I can tell you that might help. Or at least I can give you some perspective. It is this:

You cannot control whether you get pregnant.

Not at all.

Yes, I know. That probably stung a little. Also, you're reading this book because you can't get pregnant, and for heaven's sake, you're looking for a little hope! I can give you hope, if hope means, "I hope this will eventually feel better." I can give you humor, if humor means learning how to crack jokes about pelvic exams and vaginas. But no one can tell you the precise steps you need to take to have a baby.

If you feel like that's bad news, you're right.

Furthermore, I can tell you that no matter how much you *think* you know about how babies are made, you probably don't know enough. Actually, if you're anything like my husband and I were when we started this journey, what you know a lot about is how to prevent babies. How to make them is a whole different ball of wax.

As we hit "publish" on this book, Malcolm and I will both be almost forty years old. Yes, that is considered "advanced maternal age." No, we didn't start trying a year ago. We started trying when we were thirty, shortly after we got married. Or we thought we did. Really, we just stopped trying not to get pregnant. It was a while before we knew how ineffective our efforts were.

Neither of us knew how little we knew about making babies either. We like to flatter ourselves thinking that we're smart, and we both paid attention in sex-ed. Though if I'm really honest, I didn't pay quite enough attention. Health class in high school was one of the few classes I did not get an A in. I didn't think I needed to study anything I'd learned, and because I was a goody-two-shoes, I knew nothing about the slang terms for drugs other kids were smoking at the time.

If Malcolm fared better, it is because he did study, but we're both still pretty straight-laced. It's going to kill my family to hear me talking about sex so openly. (Don't worry, Mom! Most of infertility isn't about sex. This book could be graphic at times, but it will not be pornographic!)

Anyway, regardless of our sex-ed smarts, Malcolm and I did both walk out of sex-ed knowing exactly what we needed to do to prevent pregnancy. We were both highly successful with our efforts. Neither of us ever had an unplanned pregnancy. There are no abortions in our pasts. And heck, *millions* of people who aren't as academically smart as we think we are have babies every year. They pop those things out like it's easy.

Now, my husband and I had vastly different ideas when we started out about just how much work we'd have to go through to have a baby, but we did agree on one point. We thought it was reasonable to expect that we could get married at thirty, enjoy married life for a year or two, then start having kids.

The joke is on us. We're not nearly as smart as we thought. We hardly knew anything about how babies get made except that it had something to do with a sperm meeting an egg and voila!

I don't know where you are in your knowledge of how basic reproduction works, but in case you're at all like us, I'm going to go over an extremely basic primer that will not help you get pregnant but might help you with some terminology.

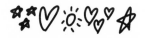

BASIC HUMAN REPRODUCTION

So how does reproduction work for a woman with a uterus and a man who produces sperm? Here are the bare-bones basics.

During their reproductive years, women typically have a menstrual cycle that prepares their body to get pregnant about once a month. In the first half of that cycle, hormones cause some eggs in the woman's ovaries (which are egg-storing, egg-growing, and hormone-producing organs) to mature. While this is happening, hormones also cause the lining of the woman's uterus (the organ that will contain a growing baby if one is created) to thicken.

About halfway through the woman's cycle, one mature egg will leave the ovary and travel through the woman's fallopian tube (an organ that connects ovary to uterus).

An egg will usually live in the fallopian tube for about 12-24 hours before it exits into the uterus, to be discarded a couple of weeks later, along with the thickened uterine lining, if it is not fertilized. The "shedding" of the unfertilized egg and uterine lining is what happens when a woman bleeds during her period. The first day of a woman's period is considered the first day of her next menstrual cycle.

But of course, we are hoping for a fertilized egg if we want to get pregnant. This requires sperm, which develop in the man's testes (which are sperm-producing, sperm-storing, and hormone-producing organs). When a man ejaculates, hordes of sperm come out of the man's penis in a fluid called semen. If the man's penis is inside a woman's vagina or close enough for semen to reach a woman's vagina when he ejaculates, the sperm in that semen will attempt to swim up the woman's vagina, through the cervix (the doorway between the vagina and the uterus), into the uterus, and then into the woman's fallopian tubes.

Sperm can survive in the uterus and fallopian tubes for about six days before they die. But if a sperm finds an egg in a woman's fallopian tube, the sperm will attempt to penetrate ("fertilize") the egg.

A fertilized egg is called a "blastocyst," and it is only a couple of cells initially. Those cells start to divide rapidly after fertilization, and the blastocyst moves from the fallopian tube into the uterus over two to three days. Once the blastocyst gets into the woman's uterus, it will try to attach to the lining of the uterus. This is called "implantation." Usually, implantation happens about six days after fertilization and can take a few days to complete.

Successful implantation is when pregnancy begins and when the uterus starts making hormones that prevent the woman from shedding that uterine lining. The hormones also tell the woman's body that she is pregnant. The blastocyst gets renamed "embryo," the cells in the embryo continue to divide, and the embryo will hopefully develop into a baby over the next thirty-six weeks or so.

If a woman gets pregnant, the first week of her menstrual cycle is considered week one of her pregnancy. Ovulation happens near the end of week two. Fertilization and implantation occur sometime during week three. By the end of week four, there are usually enough pregnancy hormones in the woman's body for a home pregnancy test to show if she is pregnant. The woman should go into labor around week forty.

That's the sex education version of human reproduction, and by the way, I used several websites to make sure I was getting most of this mostly right.[3] I highly recommend checking out some to get a sense of what information is even out there about sex-ed or trying to get pregnant if you do a basic Google search. The Scarleteen website is targeted at teenagers in particular. When you take a look, note that you would walk away from reading just about any of the articles I cited thinking that if you have unprotected sex most of the time, chances are, you'll be pregnant within a year.

TWO TRUTHS ABOUT CREATING LIFE

So here's the thing: all that sex-ed won't help you much when it comes to infertility. A young couple having a lot of unprotected sex might get pregnant pretty easily, but that doesn't mean getting pregnant is *actually* easy. It means that some people manage it without any more information than what they learned in school because they do it when they are young, super fertile, and having so much sex that they're bound to hit that lucky window of time when the woman can get pregnant at least sometimes.

However, unless you're a medical professional, you probably don't know how hard pregnancy becomes if you aren't young, super fertile, and having sex all the time. This holds true even if you've read all the books on fertility and basal body temperature charting and you paid close attention in a real anatomy class. In fact, I would take a guess and say that as a maturish adult who wants to get pregnant and is having some trouble, your knowledge of how to make babies lies somewhere between these two ideas:

Idea one: to get pregnant, a sperm has to meet an egg. A woman ovulates about two weeks after her period. So if my partner and I want to make a baby, all we have to do is have sex a few times a week every week she's not on her period. If we do this for two or three cycles, we'll probably get pregnant in a couple of months. If we don't want to get pregnant, all we have to do is use condoms and birth control to make sure a sperm never randomly meets an egg.

Idea two: to get pregnant, a sperm has to meet an egg. A woman releases an egg when she ovulates, something that happens on a cyclical basis. Also, because I really really want to get pregnant, I've read a lot of fertility books, and I know ovulation doesn't necessarily happen two weeks after the woman's period. So if my partner and I want to make a baby, we need to know exactly when she is ovulating. We can learn this by getting an ovulation kit at the drugstore, or she can track her basal body temperature religiously so that she knows more naturally when she is ovulating.

Since an egg only lives 12 to 24 hours, we will need to track her ovulation well enough to have sex a day before she ovulates, which will give his sperm time to travel up those fallopian tubes and meet that egg. If we don't want to get pregnant, all we have to do is not have sex the week before she ovulates or two days after unless we are using condoms.

Personally, I have been in both those camps, and while these ideas might hold true for someone who is not struggling with pregnancy, I now know the truth for someone who is struggling actually lies somewhere between two things that two different reproductive endocrinologists have said to me over the years.

Doctor 1: Any woman can get pregnant any time, assuming she ovulates and some sperm finds the egg.

Doctor 2: We don't always know why a woman can't get pregnant. Sometimes, it comes down to bad luck.

Here's the thing, reader. It is true that we know how a perfect reproductive cycle should theoretically work. But when you are having trouble getting pregnant, your reproductive cycles aren't perfect. Because of this, I feel pretty confident telling you that you could get pregnant any time, assuming you ovulate and some sperm finds that egg, or you could never get pregnant, and it could just be bad luck.

That is the truth. You don't know as much as you think you know about making babies because no one does.

I know that sounds intuitively wrong. After all, modern medicine is impressive. We can make artificial legs and arms, transplant hearts, livers, and kidneys, treat cancers and prevent viral infections (sometimes).

Additionally, there are all kinds of treatments you can go through to try to get pregnant. There are drugs and procedures that can work very hard together to create the optimal environment in your uterus for a baby to grow in. There are other drugs and procedures that can ensure that only top-notch embryos are being put in that perfect uterus.

Yes, your doctor might be able to put a nice, big juicy Grade A embryo that seems to be growing at the right speed and has all the right chromosomes into your beautifully prepared uterus. Then you could be pumped with all the right drugs at all the right times, and yet, that embryo might not make it. But you could go on vacation next month, randomly ovulate, have sex on the beach at exactly the right time, and get pregnant without any help at all.

No technology can predict with absolute certainty what will create a successful pregnancy. We cannot command life to be born. So as you go into this, you need to know that there is *nothing* you can do to force a life to be made in your body. There are a million reasons you might not be getting pregnant, but the only reason anyone ever *does* get pregnant is that a sperm meets an egg and a miracle occurs.

That is what having any baby is. *A miracle.* I don't care if you want to attribute (or blame) that miracle on luck or God. A baby is a miracle. The end.

INFERTILITY LESSON #2

The sooner you come to grips with the fact that you cannot control whether you get pregnant, the better.

You could go through one infertility treatment and get pregnant the first time, or you could go through twenty and never get pregnant. You, your partner, and your doctors could do everything possible to make your body the perfect receptor of life, and it might not happen.

You can't eat, breathe, exercise, meditate, or buy your way to a baby. Reducing all the stress in your life won't make it happen. Nor will having sex every day for a year, ingesting a vitamin cocktail your friend recommended, or going to the world's most incredible fertility clinic. You might *improve* your chances with those things, but nothing you do can ensure you will get pregnant.

If you are an ambitious person, this may be particularly difficult to wrap your mind around. In all other areas of your life, hard work will most often result in a predictable reward. In this area, hard work doesn't always pay off. Your work ethic, your academic talents, your intelligence, your people skills, your street smarts … none of that means squat when it comes to baby-making.

Not only that, but while you're fighting for just one baby,

you have to watch babies being born into the worst possible situations every day. Babies are born to abusive parents. Babies are abandoned and mistreated. Babies are born to drug addicts. Babies are born to parents who cannot afford to have more children. Babies are born to young, healthy women who then choose to give them up or abort them. That will hurt whether you are pro-life or pro-choice.

It is a harsh reality. As you go through this, it might even start to seem like nature has a bias in favor of stupid people who would make bad parents when it comes to reproduction. Have you seen that movie *Idiocracy*? Go watch the scene about reproduction. Try to laugh so that it won't make you cry.

This is not a "fair" process. However, if you know that now, maybe you'll be better prepared when you realize your dreams may not come true. It will still suck to be the victim of an unfair process. But then, life isn't fair, is it? No one controls who dies young, who gets cancer, who wins the lotto. Why would we expect the creation of life to be any fairer than any other aspect of life?

Reset your expectations and check your assumptions. I am so sorry, but you cannot control whether you will ever get pregnant and have babies. Start coping with that now.

INFERTILITY IS A MOVING TARGET

There's one more thing you need to know about this. In addition to the fact that pregnancy isn't predictable or fair, you will find that your own infertility is a moving target.

I took one of those magazine quizzes a couple of years ago about infertility. It was titled something like, "How much do you really know about infertility?" I got every question right, and my "results" said something like, "You must be an ob/gyn to know so much."

No kidding.

Despite that, I have found that there is always something new to learn. For example, I thought for years that the only reason I couldn't get pregnant is that I hardly ever had periods. I assumed this was PCOS, and eventually, someone did confirm that diagnosis for me. But surprise! I also have adenomyosis, which is similar to endometriosis and can make it harder to get pregnant.

One of the mistakes I see other women make with infertility is that they try to control the situation by identifying exactly the problem preventing them from getting pregnant. That instinct is understandable, but it's based on flawed logic. It assumes that you can *ever* identify one specific reason that you aren't getting pregnant.

What happened to me? Why couldn't I get pregnant? Was it my PCOS? My adenomyosis? A combination of the two problems? Something else? Something we never learned about my husband? Just poor luck? I'll never know.

And to put some icing on this, you will find that there are problems that crop up as you age, new obstacles to overcome, things that were never discovered before. That means that even if I can identify every reason I can't get pregnant right this second, those reasons could change tomorrow.

I believe in doing your best to learn what's going on with your own body. It is good to know if there are things you can do to increase your chances of getting pregnant. But while you're trying to figure yourself out, do it with the understanding that this isn't a static situation. The minute you think you understand what's going on and how to fix it, things will change. Best to learn how to go with the flow.

<u>FINAL THOUGHTS ON MAKING BABIES</u>

One of my friends going through this years ago put the whole crux of the problem to me like this: to have a baby, the sun, the moon, and all the stars have to align. She was not wrong. When you see a baby, stop and be awed for a moment. Not just because the baby is cute but because the *entire universe* had to move for that baby to be born.

As long as you and I aren't in charge of the entire universe, the creation of life is ultimately out of our hands. Life is a true miracle. All you can do is work with a good doctor to try to increase your odds. After that, it's all up to fate.

CHAPTER THREE
What Men Don't Know

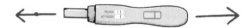

FAMILY PLANNING

It is 2011, I'm twenty-nine years old, I am engaged to the man who will become my husband, and we are currently driving to Michigan to visit our parents. Also, we are having an enormous fight. Because I want to talk about kids, and he wants to talk about the motorcycle he just bought. Our conversation is going something like this:

Me: "I want to have four kids. This is important to me. If you don't want kids, I need to know before we get married."

Him: "I don't see why we need to decide *now* to have four kids. Why can't we just start with one and see what happens?"

Me: "But I *definitely* want more than one kid. Kids need siblings. I don't want an only child. That would be so lonely."

Him: "*I* am an only child. I was fine. I don't see why we can't start with one and see how it goes."

Me: "But it's a possibility you'll want more than one, right? You're not ruling out more? Because I want four, so I think we shouldn't wait very long to start."

Him: "We aren't even *thirty* yet! No one else my age at my firm has kids. Why do we have to worry about this now?"

Me: "Because I'm worried it will be hard for us to have children! And if we *do* want to have more than one, I don't want to wait until I'm in my late thirties to start! That will make us old parents, and I don't want to be old parents! We'll have less energy. Our kids will have less time with us. They'll have less time with their grandparents."

Him: "My mom was thirty-eight when she had me. That worked out fine."

Me: "*Except* that you act like you were born in the fifties!"

Him: "You're just freaking out because your parents are pressuring you to have kids."

Me: "THEY ARE NOT! Me not wanting to be an old parent has nothing to do with whether my parents want grandchildren. And I'm allowed to want my kids to have time with their grandparents. And your parents are older than mine, so why aren't you worried about this?"

Him: "I don't see why we have to worry. Why can't we just get married and then stop trying to prevent children at some point and see what happens?"

Me: "I DO NOT HAVE PERIODS. We aren't going to randomly have children by not trying to prevent them!"

Him: "This is ridiculous. We are too young to plan our family right now. I'm confident that my swimmers are good. I'm sure when we want kids, we can just have a lot of sex, and we'll get pregnant. Also, I'm thinking of trading my motorcycle in for something faster and more dangerous."

The conversation devolves into shouting and arguing, and we do not resolve the issue. I decide that maybe I *am*

panicking. We do have plenty of time, right? Even if we ultimately have to do IVF? We aren't even married yet. When
we get married, we will barely be thirty. And he's not saying
he doesn't want multiple children. He's saying he doesn't see
why we should even be thinking past a first baby when we
aren't ready for kids yet anyway.

This will not be the only time we have a version of this
fight, though. We will have the fight again shortly after we're
married and again after we stop trying to prevent children.

We will *still* be having the fight a few years later when
we make an appointment at a fertility clinic for the first time.
It will take five years, and *many* infertility treatments, before
Malcolm realizes that he is now one of the only men in his
peer group who does not have children. Then it will dawn
on him that we may *never* have children. He will know more,
too, so he will know that the one son he wanted to start with
would have been much easier to get if we hadn't delayed so
much after we got married.

But you can't roll back time, and I will turn out to be
right on this one. He will end up regretting not taking me
more seriously when I told him I thought we needed to enlist
help early to get pregnant.

What will I regret? That when we had those early
conversations, I over-focused on how *many* children I wanted
and under-focused on the vast difference between what he
knew and what I knew about my ability to get pregnant.

I sincerely wish I had set up a consultation with a reproductive endocrinologist immediately after we got married.
That would have put my husband and me on the same page
far earlier. Maybe we would have started egg retrievals and
diagnostic tests immediately, even if we delayed IVF for a
while. Though maybe we would have started treatments and

still not had any success for years. The point is, we would have known more about what we were up against.

What else will I regret? Making my husband feel like he was to blame for those early delays. We both made choices that delayed our progress. In some ways, this is on me. I knew better. He truly didn't.

FREQUENTLY ASKED QUESTION

My spouse says his "swimmers" are fine and we don't need to worry about getting pregnant until our mid-thirties. We're in our early thirties now, so I know we have plenty of time left. Still, I have PCOS and I don't get regular periods. Is my husband right? Am I just being paranoid?

ANSWER: YOUR HUSBAND IS WRONG

Infertility is a major pitfall for couples. This is especially true if your infertility treatments are unsuccessful. A big Danish study found that women who don't have a child after infertility treatments are three times more likely to divorce or end living with their partner than those who do.[4] Another review of multiple infertility studies found that infertile women were more likely than fertile women to have a less stable marital relationship.[5] And a Stanford study found that women with infertility were at higher risk for sexual dysfunction compared to women without infertility.[6]

Yep. Infertility is hard on a marriage.

I would, of course, love to tell you that my marriage was never troubled by infertility, but that would be a big lie.

Malcolm and I had all kinds of fights about babies, mostly stemming from one big problem, which was our very different knowledge about reproduction.

Neither of us had it right in the beginning. As you've already seen from Chapter Two, I believed that if I could get to the right doctor and get the right treatment at the right time, then I could have those four kids I wanted, spaced out exactly as I wanted them. I had a plan, and I thought I had this all under my control. I was so wrong.

Malcolm did not have the same issue with obsessively wanting kids and thinking he could control when we had them. Where he got it wrong was thinking we could just relax and trust that all the pieces would fall into place if we just had sex like a normal couple.

He genuinely thought I was crazy to be worried about reproduction before we were even married, except to the extent that we did not want children before marriage. Then he thought I was paranoid to be worried about it in our early thirties. But there is a massive gender gap when it comes to what men and women know about getting pregnant. He had no way of knowing how wrong he was.

Maybe this is because reproductive problems are more obvious to women early on. We, women, have to contend with our reproductive systems for years—sometimes decades—before we ever start wanting to reproduce. If you are a woman and your spouse or partner is male, this means you had to face your own reproductive health *far* earlier than your spouse did.

Think about it this way. When you have a uterus, you hit puberty in your very early teenage years and start having to worry about periods, menstrual cramps, and PMS right then. You may have to begin seeing a gynecologist annually so that someone can stick a speculum up your vag and conduct a pap smear before you've ever even had sex.

Then sex becomes a whole thing, and you have all kinds of misconceptions to freak out over related to your reproductive system. Can you get pregnant if you "do it" while you're on your period? Is there really some mythical barrier called a hymen that's going to "pop" or "break" the first time you have sex? If so, will it hurt? Will all your future sexual partners know if you've done it before?

And omg, what about STDs, yeast infections, and UTIs, not to mention all those birth control choices?! Should you start on the pill? The patch? Get an IUD? Just use condoms? Where do you get any of that from? A doctor? A pharmacy? What should you do if a boy you want to have sex with doesn't want to use condoms? Are you willing to have sex without condoms if you're on the pill?

Then God forbid you ever have an accident! If that condom broke or he promised he would "pull out" but didn't quite make it on time, then *you* were the one who had to decide if you were going to make a late-night run to get the Plan B pill. If your period was late, you were also the one who had to buy a pregnancy test, pee on a stick, and wait, wondering if your life was about to change forever, and not in a good way.

If you did get pregnant, you then had to decide what to do about it. Maybe you had a baby and had to give it up. Maybe you had an abortion. Maybe you were raped or sexually assaulted. All those things happened in and to *your* body.

But even if you never went through anything traumatic related to an unwanted pregnancy, you still had things to worry about. You could have been completely abstinent and then had to worry about your period stopping entirely or starting and never stopping for reasons you didn't understand. You might always have used proper protection and never have had a pregnancy scare, and yet, sex could have become incredibly painful for you. Those events would have meant you had to go to a doctor to get help. Which means you had to have an adult conversation about your reproductive organs when you were very young.

Basically: if you have a uterus, your reproductive health has been up in your face since you were twelve. Maybe you didn't know until just recently how hard it could be to get pregnant, and a lot of what you know about your own body could be based on misconceptions. But you still have a lot of knowledge. If you have a reason to think you might not be able to get pregnant, that is enough for me to feel quite confident telling you that yes, it would be worth your time and money to see a doctor and get some real facts.

Now, do you know what your partner knows about reproduction? Assuming your partner is male? Let me sum it up for you. Your male partner knows:

1. How to get off.

2. How to tell a dirty joke.

3. How to put on a condom. (Mostly. He still gets this wrong sometimes, especially when he's in a rush.)

My husband would add that beyond that lack of reproductive knowledge, most guys—or at least most guys like him—spent their teenage years and early twenties terrified of getting some girl pregnant. He assumed that if he had sex, even once, without condoms, pregnancy was an inevitability.

This wasn't some trumped-up toxic masculinity assumption, either. This was him being reasonably afraid of a life-changing possibility that could have completely derailed his education and career. Also, if an eighteen-year-old guy has sex with his healthy girlfriend without a condom, and she's not on any birth control, then yeah, there's a pretty decent chance he could get her pregnant.

Now, can we blame that same guy for later thinking that getting his own wife pregnant would be easy?

Come on. How the hell was he supposed to know that the strength of his "swimmers" was only one tiny little factor in this whole equation? Periods have always been mysterious for him! He's spent *years* focused solely on preventing his swimmers from getting anywhere near you! *Of course,* he's going to assume that you'll get pregnant the minute you stop using condoms. *That's how we taught him to think!*

There are a lot of things you'll have to do to keep your marriage or partnership strong while you go through infertility challenges, but you can do yourself a big favor right here by assuming that you and your male partner do not come at this problem from the same angle. Yep. You probably know more than he does about how your ovaries work.

INFERTILITY LESSON #3

You and your partner may have very different ideas about how easy or hard it will be to get pregnant. You should talk about this early to find out how far apart you are. The potential discrepancy between what you and your partner know about your ability to reproduce is a great reason to see a reproductive endocrinologist early if one of you thinks you might have trouble getting pregnant.

If your partner is concerned that you're starting far too early, and you feel you're not, maybe this is the time for some couples counseling. Because this is one of those areas where it's quite difficult just to talk things out, and handing a book about infertility to your partner might not be enough to convince him that you're right about this.

Keep in mind that you both have years and years of societal programming and life experience telling you what is "true" about reproduction. **Your male spouse isn't trying to be an egotistical asshat when he tells you he's sure that just having a lot of sex is all you need to get pregnant. He believes that. It's a core belief, even.**

And if you're a man reading this, and your female partner is telling you she's sure she's going to have problems getting pregnant, please do not assume she's pushing the panic button on having kids. Trust me when I tell you that simply walking into a fertility clinic is not a way to get pregnant. It is a way to help you do some real family planning.

FINAL THOUGHTS ON THE GENDER GAP

It is incredibly emotionally draining when you can't get pregnant, and that takes a toll on any relationship. You don't want to start this journey fighting about things you can easily resolve. There are all kinds of options out there for couples who want to have babies, are worried they won't be able to have them easily, but still think they are a bit young for kids. Get that information, and maybe neither of you will ever have to regret things you did and said that prevented you from planning early enough.

PART II
At the Fertility Clinic

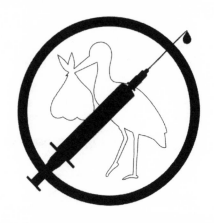

I think it's the worst thing that we do to each other as women, not share the truth about our bodies and how they work, and how they don't work.
~ Michelle Obama

CHAPTER FOUR
Diagnostic Delays (Fertility Testing)

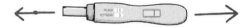

WAITING OUT A COLD SWEAT

It is spring 2014, I'm thirty-two, and my husband and I have finally made it to a fertility clinic. It's been almost two years since I first started having conversations with doctors about my fertility, so I feel like I've waited long enough already. I'm eager to get started with "real" infertility treatments, which I assume is in vitro fertilization (IVF).

I am immediately disappointed. The only thing we can start right away is bloodwork, and there's a lot of bloodwork to be done. First, the clinic tests my antimüllerian hormone (AMH), follicle-stimulating hormone (FSH), and estradiol to make sure my "ovarian reserve" is sufficient.

The number of eggs a woman has decreases as she ages, along with egg quality. So one reason some women have trouble getting pregnant is that their "ovarian reserve" isn't high enough, or, in normal person terms, they don't have enough eggs left.[7] Low ovarian reserve equates to low pregnancy rates, but based on my bloodwork, my ovarian reserve appears to be fine.

The clinic also takes blood for carrier screening from both my husband and me. Carrier screening is genetic screening that determines whether you or your spouse are likely to carry the genes for a disorder like cystic fibrosis or sickle cell disease. Whether you need specific carrier screening is sometimes determined by your family history or your ethnic background.[8] Malcolm and I do not test positive for anything. So far, so good.

Since I don't have periods, the doctor adds thyroid tests to my bloodwork. My thyroid-stimulating hormone (TSH) is a little low, and that can also affect fertility[9], so the doctor prescribes Synthroid to bring my TSH levels back up.

Initially, I think that's quite a lot of bloodwork. But fertility clinics need more blood than vampires. During a typical infertility cycle, the clinic usually draws my blood at least four times, sometimes more. I am very thankful to have good veins, and I always feel bad when I am sitting next to a woman in the lab whose veins are difficult to find. Ladies, stay hydrated! You're going to want your veins to be easy to find.

Unfortunately, other than the bloodwork, none of the diagnostic tests the fertility clinic wants to run can start immediately. Well, that's not totally true. My husband's semen analysis can happen at any time. But for me, diagnostic testing revolves around the timing of my menstrual cycle, and the one thing I know is interfering with my ability to get pregnant is my mostly non-existent menstrual cycle. How do you know what day of your menstrual cycle you're on if you never get periods?

Turns out, the solution is to go back on birth control for a few weeks, stop the birth control, wait for my period to start (birth control makes me have periods), and then call the clinic to let them know my period has started. This is an incredible frustration for me. My stupid lack of periods delays starting the diagnostic testing for several weeks, and I feel like that's a long time.

I have a lot to learn.

I go through those weeks of birth control, wait for my period to start, and then the testing can finally begin. First, there's a saline ultrasound, also called a "saline infusion sono-hysterography" (SIS or SHG).[10] The saline ultrasound is where I start discovering what the "poking" and "prodding" of infertility feels like.

Spoiler alert: it feels bad.

To perform the saline ultrasound, the doctor inserts a speculum into my vagina, just like a doctor would for a normal ob/gyn exam. He widens the speculum so he can get to my cervix, then he threads a little tube through my cervix and pumps saline through the tube and into my uterus. The threading hurts, and I cramp up when they pump the saline in. (Cramping is typical for this procedure. I am not uniquely sensitive about pain.)

While the saline, tube, and speculum are all still in place, the doctor performs an ultrasound to look at my uterus, uterine lining, and ovaries. There is nothing abnormal about my parts. At least not today.

The tools are removed, and I'm still cramped. The nurse recommends Motrin for pain. I feel like I've just had a pap smear on steroids, and also, I feel like I'm kind of a martyr in my own house for having gone through that.

I'm so so naïve. The saline ultrasound is a test I'll have to repeat several times over the years, and I won't flinch at it later. It turns out to be the easiest of all the tests I'll ever have to do involving a speculum.

The next diagnostic test is a hysterosalpingogram (HSG), and it's performed another day. For this procedure, they tell me to take Motrin in advance, which should probably tell me something about the test.

The HSG is similar to the saline ultrasound at first. There's a speculum, a tube is threaded through my cervix, and then an iodine solution is pumped into my uterus. But the iodine must be thicker than the saline because it hurts worse. I have to do this test while I'm lying under an enormous x-ray machine, and that gives the doctor a look at my uterus, ovaries, and fallopian tubes.[11]

Malcolm isn't allowed in the room for this. They tell me it's because the x-ray machine takes up too much space for an additional person to fit in the room. I later think it's because they don't want your partner panicking while tears spring to your eyes. Thankfully, the test only takes a couple of minutes, and then it's over. The nurse tells me to expect some cramping to continue and some fluid to leak out. I complain about the HSG as we drive home and feel like even *more* of a martyr. But at least the tests are over. For a while.

Fast forward to January 2015. I'm thirty-three now, and after several failed timed intercourse and IUI cycles (more on those in the next chapter), we're getting ready for IVF. By now, I am aware that there is *always* more testing available, and today, I'm lying on a table in a cold room, waiting for another to begin.

Today's test is a diagnostic hysteroscopy.[12] Malcolm wasn't available to bring me to the clinic, so my aunt drove me instead. But I'm alone in the room with the doctor and a nurse. There is a video monitor in the room, too, and there's a large tray of instruments sitting near the examination table.

A blue paper towel covers the instruments, and the room seems quiet. The doctor already has the speculum in place, but there's been some kind of delay. So he's sitting at the end of the exam table looking grumpy and awkward while I try to tolerate the combination of excessive stretching and pinching that always comes with a speculum.

The nurse uncovers that tray of tools, and I see something that looks kind of like an extremely long knitting needle. I think it must be at least eighteen inches long, and *this* is the tube the doctor will thread up my cervix and into my uterus for this procedure. There's a little camera at the end of the tube, and the doctor will use the camera to look around my uterus on the video screen.

The doctor inserts the tube. It is painful. Much more painful than I remember either the saline ultrasound or the HSG test being. I tell myself not to freak out. They do this all the time. It's going to be over soon, right? Except, then the video equipment won't work. So now the speculum is stretching and pinching me, the tube is hurting me, and the doctor looks even grouchier and more awkward as he and the nurse communicate about the malfunctioning video monitor.

The nurse leaves the room to find someone else to come and fix the monitor. This seems to take forever, and in the meanwhile, I'm trying to breathe and not panic while it all starts to get to me. This kind of discomfort is not the surprise kind that makes you cry suddenly. This is sustained pain, and the fact that the test hasn't even technically started yet is raising my anxiety levels. Cold sweat starts to form on my neck and back, and I fight my body while it begins to shake. I know shaking won't make this better.

I make a light joke to try to reduce my anxiety. "I guess this is probably nothing compared to labor pains, right?" Ha ha ha.

The doctor kind of grunts at me. What does that mean? Does it mean he thinks it is ridiculous for me even to consider the comparison? As in: "Lady, labor is so bad that you'll wish you were just doing a hysteroscopy while you're going through that." Or is he grunting because this *is* that bad? Does he even know? This is a male doctor. He doesn't have a cervix. For all I know, that grunt just means he's ticked off that he's stuck here for ten minutes longer than he wanted to be today.

They finally get the video monitor working, and they proceed with the test. When it is over, the doctor tells me my uterus is "heart-shaped," but he does not think this is a problem causing my infertility. I try to hide that I'm still shaking all over as I listen to him and then leave the office, but I'm glad I had my aunt bring me here. The drive home is through Atlanta interstate traffic, and I'm upset enough that I wouldn't be a good driver right now.

In early 2018, another doctor at the same clinic casually suggests repeating the hysteroscopy. Your uterus can change quite a lot over even a single year. I tell her I don't think I can handle the pain, and that's when I find out that a hysteroscopy can be done under anesthesia, but the anesthesia makes the test much more expensive.

We have a high-deductible insurance plan that year, and it covers some infertility procedures. I try to find out what the cost of the hysteroscopy would be if we do it with anesthesia, but no one can tell me for sure. Apparently, my insurance company is a little random about what it covers in terms of anesthesia and an operating room. The hysteroscopy will cost somewhere between $750 and $5000 out-of-pocket if we do it with anesthesia.

I am stressed about this, and the doctor doesn't seem to

think the hysteroscopy is absolutely necessary, so I decide I'm not signing up to repeat a test that hurt like hell the first time and might now cost thousands and thousands of dollars.

After that, our lives and our infertility treatments are interrupted. My husband takes a new job in Raleigh, North Carolina, and we have to move away from Atlanta, Georgia. We get set up with a new fertility clinic in Raleigh several months later. I have to repeat a saline ultrasound in early 2019, and during that procedure, my new doctor notices what he thinks might be scar tissue and recommends that we do a hysteroscopy.

I can't imagine what my face looks like when he says that. I start protesting. "If we're going to do this, I at least need Xanax or something," I tell the new doctor.

"Oh, you'll be out for the hysteroscopy," the doctor says, as if it isn't even a question. "We don't do these procedures in our office. We do them at a surgery center with anesthesia. You shouldn't feel anything during the procedure."

I end up having three hysteroscopy procedures in total during my infertility journey. What I remember most vividly about the first hysteroscopy is that cold sweat. What I remember about the others is that operating rooms are kind of bright, and it's a little awkward to slide your butt to the end of a table and put your legs into stirrups while three or four people are milling around you. But after that, the anesthesia always kicks in, and I'm a fan of anesthesia.

Still, in my personal hell, I'm waiting for an infertility cycle to begin, and while I wait, a doctor is rotating me through a never-ending train of diagnostic tests. I have my blood drawn, then I go in for a saline ultrasound, then an HSG, then a hysteroscopy (without anesthesia), then a mock embryo cycle with a uterine biopsy and endometrial receptivity analysis[13] (the worst of the lot, in my opinion, and something I'll get to in later chapters).

So, you thought you'd just get an appointment and start IVF next week? Well, maybe you'll get luckier than I did.

Maybe.

FREQUENTLY ASKED QUESTION

I booked an appointment with a reproductive endocrinologist. They couldn't get me in until the end of the month, and now I'm worried that means I won't be able to start treatments right away. I feel so behind. How long until we get to the "two-week wait?"

ANSWER: THE TWO-WEEK WAIT IS NOTHING

As I begin to write this part of the chapter, and to answer this question, I am talking to my husband about cars. Malcolm likes stuff that goes fast. Motor sports are his thing. He fantasizes about drifting cars around corners and driving curvy, twisty roads that make me carsick. I rent us affordable sedans for our vacations, and he "negotiates" with the rental car companies while I'm not looking so he can drive convertibles in California.

He is ridiculously proud of the number of times he's driven Tail of the Dragon, which is this insanely loopy, mountainous road that car guys like Malcolm drool over. I *still* consider the day he finally sold his last motorcycle, a Kawasaki crotch rocket, to be the day I knew he'd survive into his thirties.

Point being: I married a guy who does not do slow. But I will admit that this little problem is both one of our biggest fights and also his most endearing flaw. Secretly, I'm a car girl, and I like things that go fast, too. God knows I didn't want to marry a golfer. Malcolm earned his second date by picking me up in a Jaguar for our first date. So, if my husband tends to conveniently misunderstand when I ask him to slow down on the curves, I brought that on myself.

Since it is fair to say that neither my husband nor I are people who naturally enjoy waiting for things, you can imagine how anxious we were to get started when it came to infertility treatments. We were then floored by the amount of waiting we had to do, right from the get-go.

This is something no one understands about infertility before they actually start seeing a doctor. The hell of infertility isn't just about your deep desire to have children, your fear that you will never have children, or your grief over every embryo that does not materialize into a baby. It's not just about the treatments themselves or all the monitoring and medication.

There's also all the waiting and delays. There are the tests you didn't know you needed. There's your period not starting when it was supposed to or your body needing five extra days of medication to ovulate. There's your fertility clinic not being able to schedule your next cycle until after the holidays.

You need the patience of a saint to get through infertility, and if you don't have that patience initially, you will when it's over. *Everything* about infertility is a waiting game.

Compare to what a "normal" couple goes through to get pregnant. First, the couple has sex a few times during the middle of the woman's cycle, which is only about 28 days long. Then, they wait two weeks for the woman's next period to begin.

If her period starts, they know she's not pregnant, and now they can roll right into another "try." But if her period doesn't start, they can purchase a home pregnancy test at the drugstore. They'll take that test home, she'll pee on it, they'll wait two minutes, and that's how long it will take to find out if she's pregnant. If they get lucky, they'll get that BFP (slang for "big fat positive," which means "positive pregnancy test") the very first time.

The two weeks that couple waits between when they have sex and when her period starts is affectionately called the "Two Week Wait" on the Internet, where you can find a plethora of whiny women complaining about how they *just can't han•le* the suspense of the Two Week Wait. It is *so har•* to wait fourteen whole days to see if your period will start again. It is *so awful* when "Aunt Flo" (your period) comes anyway. It is so *incre•ibly horribly har•* when you have to do this six or seven times before you get pregnant.

But despite the whining, most couples get that BFP within a year from when they first start trying. The woman misses her period. She pees on a stick. Two lines show up on the test. Hurrah! She's pregnant! They plan a gender reveal party that will hopefully not start a rampant wildfire in California.

That is not *at all* how it works for a couple going through infertility. For starters, most people dealing with infertility "try" to get pregnant for at least a year before they get frustrated and find a doctor.

Wait #1: the year or more it takes before you know you need help getting pregnant.

Once you realize you need help getting pregnant, you'll have to research doctors in your area, find a fertility clinic, call up the clinic, and schedule an initial consult with a reproductive endocrinologist. Every doctor is different, but based on our experience with two separate clinics, you should expect your first consult to take two-to-four weeks to schedule.

Wait #2: the two-to-four weeks it takes to get in and see a doctor for the first time.

During the consultation, the doctor will talk to you about your history, and they will recommend a battery of diagnostic tests. They might be able to do one or two of the tests at the consult, but probably that will only be bloodwork. The rest of the tests—which could include anything from simple pelvic ultrasounds to a uterine biopsy—probably won't be done the same day you see the doctor for the first time. That's because most of these tests have to occur at certain times in your cycle. You'll need to wait for your next period to begin so that the clinic knows when to schedule your tests. If you don't get regular periods, you may have to start birth control first so that you will get a period. They will start the testing calendar around your period.

Those diagnostic tests will be your first foray into the time and money suck that infertility can be. Hopefully, your insurance will cover some of the costs. But speaking of that, your fertility clinic may also require you to make a separate appointment with their finance department and submit information about your insurance before you get started on anything big. Scheduling the financial interview will be another delay.

Wait #3: the two-to-six weeks it could take to get all those diagnostic tests done.

Finally, the doctor will have enough information to recommend an initial course of action, and you'll learn then that there are lots of different types of infertility treatments.

I'll give you the rundown of all the infertility treatments we did in the next few chapters. For now, it's probably safe to say that you could be starting with something "simple"—like drugs that will make you ovulate and timed sex—or you could be doing something much more complicated—like egg retrieval, genetic testing of the embryos, and a frozen embryo transfer.

Depending on what your doctor recommends, your first real infertility treatment cycle could take four-to-eight additional weeks to get through. Though maybe you will get super lucky and be able to start an infertility cycle while you are also doing your diagnostic testing.

Alternatively, it could take *months* to get from your initial consult to your very first pregnancy test. The longest it ever took us was about a year. That year, our initial consult was in August, we did tests in September and October, egg retrieval and genetic testing of embryos in November, break for the holidays (because fertility clinics don't like scheduling things at the end of December), more tests in January, a three-month drug treatment to try to make my uterus a more conducive place for an embryo to implant, and then, finally, a frozen transfer cycle in July.

After all that, we got a negative pregnancy test. So...

Wait #4: two weeks to an entire year for one single "try" at getting pregnant. If you got pregnant, great. But if not ...

Wait #5: two-to-four weeks to schedule the beginning of your next infertility treatment cycle.

Unfortunately, this is all best-case scenario. If you get pregnant and then later miscarry, you must also add the time during which you were pregnant and then the time it takes to recover from the miscarriage before you can try again.

Your doctor will likely want you to wait at least one full cycle before you start another infertility treatment, but you may need more time than that emotionally. After my first miscarriage, it took about two years before I was ready to start again. After my second miscarriage, we scheduled the next cycle as soon as possible, and that took about four months.

Bonus Wait: months to years to recover from a miscarriage.

So think about all that wait time. A normal couple can "try" to get pregnant ten-to-twelve times in one year. A normal couple with infertility has to "try" for six months to a year before they even get to a fertility clinic.

Then they go into the clinic feeling super anxious and stressed about how long they've been trying unsuccessfully to get pregnant. They know they're on a biological clock. They wanted to be pregnant forever ago, and they're not looking for any delays now. But they soon find out they have to do all these damn tests before they can do anything else. The tests are uncomfortable and sometimes even painful, and they can have troubling results.

All that usually has to happen before the couple can even start something like IVF, and sometimes additional testing happens between unsuccessful cycles. A couple dealing with infertility is fortunate if they get four tries in one year. A couple struggling a lot might only get one try in a year.

One try. Per year.

If you're on this journey, and you think a two-week wait sounds bad, the real deal will sound horrible. So, you don't just need pain management to get through this. You need patience. The only good thing is that pain management and patience are related. How are you going to handle this? Here's my recommendation:

INFERTILITY LESSON #4

Settle in for the long haul, reset your expectations, and start practicing patience now. This is a great time to get into mindfulness and meditation.

Find a therapist who specializes in mindfulness or go to a meditation retreat. Start attending a yin yoga class. Take your dog for long walks. Make hiking a hobby or pick up a crafty project that you can't finish in an afternoon.

Do whatever you need to do to learn how to wait. This is especially important if you've had trouble sitting still with yourself before. It could be *years* before you get that baby you want, if you ever get him or her. In the meanwhile, you have to live your life. So it can only benefit you to know how to live in the moment without over-focusing on the anxiety you have about how things will ultimately turn out.

As for the physical pain infertility could bring? There's great news there. The same skills you need to be patient, to live in the moment, and to stop your anxiety in its tracks are the skills you need to alleviate your physical pain when you're lying on a table with a long needle threaded through your cervix.

You need to be able to take a deep breath.

You need to be able to loosen up your muscles.

You need to be able to take your mind somewhere else.

You need to stop your own panic.

You need to allow your body to be out of your control without losing your mind.

So your job right now, at the beginning of your journey, is to take that list of skills you need to your therapist, your meditation leader, your favorite yoga instructor, or whoever, and tell him or her that these are the things your friend, Sandy, recommends you learn so that you can tolerate all the delays and discomforts of infertility.

But *exceptional* news: the ability to relax and have some patience when you are in pain or panic is an incredible skill to have in a stressed-the-hell-out society like ours. Knowing how simply to be still and breathe will serve you well throughout your life. Might even make you live longer.[14]

Oh, but there *is* one thing you shouldn't wait on.

If your best bottle of wine is something that needs to be opened a few years after it was bottled, don't save that particular bottle for a positive pregnancy test. You don't want that beautiful Malbec to turn to vinegar, do you? No. Drink that wine now! Consider it part of learning how to live in the moment. You're welcome.

FINAL THOUGHTS ON THE WAIT GAME

When Malcolm and I talk about all we've been through with infertility, we agree that the delays and the unknowns are some of the most difficult things.

After we had our first miscarriage, we were both very sad. Malcolm had purchased his first vintage car the year before, I think partly as a distraction for himself. It was a convertible Triumph Spitfire from 1978, and the engine in that car might have been less powerful than the engines in a lot of go-karts. The 1974 Triumph TR-6 he later purchased was a huge step up.

The '78 Spitfire had a canvas top, but the top wasn't exactly functional. We only ever drove it with the top down. It had no airbags. Malcolm had to install seat belts. It made an awful noise as we drove it out of the neighborhood that made it sound like we'd be lucky to make it back alive.

Still, about the only time I don't get carsick is when I can see all the way out of the car, and I spent hours with Malcolm in that Spitfire after the miscarriage. I would sit in the passenger seat while Malcolm drove us down little, low-traffic roads under canopies of fall leaves. I'd tip my head back, look up at the trees and the blue skies, and listen to music, and when I did that, life would seem okay. There would be more appointments to come, more waiting, more pokes and prods, more grief. But as long as we were driving (leisurely!) down an old dirt road together, we could suspend everything that hurt and just breathe in the fresh air for a while.

It's impossible to say how long your infertility journey will take or what you might be up against. Because of this, you *must* be capable of turning off the part of you that wants to skip to the chapter in your story where you have a baby. So figure out what can make you happy at this moment. Find your equivalent to a Triumph Spitfire. There are times in your life when things will go fast. This is not that time. Might as well find a way to enjoy it.

CHAPTER FIVE
Body On Display (Timed Sex & IUI)

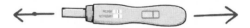

THE FIRST CYCLE

It is still spring of 2014, and my husband and I are talking to the doctor about all those diagnostic tests. I have plenty of eggs left, and my husband's sperm count is normal. My fallopian tubes are clear, and there's nothing wrong with my uterus. As far as everyone can tell, the only reason I'm not getting pregnant is that I'm not ovulating.

I would like the doctor to confirm that my lack of ovulation is because I have polycystic ovarian syndrome (PCOS).[15] I still don't have a formal diagnosis. When I was a teenager and my periods didn't start, my mother took me to a gynecologist, who put me on birth control to fix the problem and told me to return when I needed help getting pregnant.

That was nearly twenty years ago, and until I wanted to get pregnant, I mostly just stayed on birth control. I did try going off a few times, usually with disastrous consequences. Without birth control, I have unwanted hair on my face and not enough hair on my head. I get bad migraine headaches and bad acne, but not periods. From what I've read on the Internet, PCOS is the likely cause.

But my reproductive endocrinologist doesn't think I'm a clear case. "Most women with PCOS struggle with weight, acne, unwanted hair..." he tells me.

As he says this, I'm thinking about how much I've struggled. How I've always been chunky. How I always crave sugar. How I had to get laser treatments for the hair on my legs, but I still have to shave every single day if I don't want a five o'clock shadow on my inner thighs by mid-afternoon. How I've had adult acne at least twice, always off birth control, and how it's left scars all over my face.

"I, uh, feel like I've struggled with my weight," I say.

The doctor says, "It could be much worse."

Maybe this is where my slide into the indignity of infertility begins. Everything is laid bare when you're dealing with infertility. Everything. You're completely exposed for strangers to poke, prod, analyze, diagnose, and experiment on with treatments that may or may not work. A gazillion medical professionals get to know things that you have kept private for decades, and they can say things about your weight like, "It could be worse," with a straight face.

Despite the doctor's refusal to officially diagnose me with PCOS, he still thinks my problem is ovulation. He suggests that we start our first infertility treatment cycle with "timed intercourse" and a medication called Clomid, that will supposedly make me ovulate.

I stop taking my birth control pills and call the nurse as soon as my period begins. After that, I start going in for "baseline" and "monitoring" appointments. These appointments are basically the same from a patient perspective, except the "baseline" is the first of the appointments and "monitoring" is everything after. At both types of appointments, two things usually happen. There's bloodwork, and there's a transvaginal pelvic ultrasound.[16]

During a transvaginal pelvic ultrasound, a wand that looks like a long, skinny, stiff dildo is inserted into your vagina. (No. It's not at all sexy.) Usually, the wand is already set up in the exam room when you come in for the appointment. You see it there with a condom covering it and some jelly on top, connected to an ultrasound machine, as the nurse takes you into the room.

The nurse usually tells you to empty your bladder in the connected bathroom, undress from the waist down, sit on the exam table, and cover yourself with the provided sheet while you wait for the doctor. You do this, and it never gets less annoying that the paper sheet barely seems to cover your thighs.

The doctor who comes in to see you on any given day sits down at a stool in front of you, puts on gloves, and, if you're new, they might tell you to scoot forward until your butt is at the edge. You try to widen your knees an appropriate amount so that you feel cooperative but not lewd.

The doctor spreads the flaps of your vagina apart with their fingers and pushes the ultrasound wand inside you. A good doctor will make it fast and do it with some confidence, knowing that your vagina is meant to stretch. Other doctors will make it slow, like maybe it will hurt you less or you won't notice it happening if they're gentle. (Doctors, don't do that! Having something pushed slowly up your vagina only increases the amount of time you're left to think about it. Fast is much better.)

Now the wand is inside you, and the doctor moves it

around to look at your left ovary, your right ovary, your uterus, the lining of your uterus. It's uncomfortable, obviously, but not painful, and you can usually watch what they're seeing on a monitor. So the thing that sucks the most about all this is the invasion of privacy.

For our first infertility cycle, I go in for my "baseline" appointment, then I get a call in the afternoon from a nurse. She says my hormone levels are good and tells me when I should start taking Clomid. I return for another monitoring appointment a week or so later, and it's the same drill. Transvaginal pelvic ultrasound. Bloodwork.

They tell me to start using an ovulation kit, but the kit doesn't seem to work for me. It never shows that I'm ovulating. That's okay. That's what those monitoring appointments are for. Based on the monitoring appointments, the clinic finally decides I am ovulating soon, and then they tell me exactly when and how many times my husband and I are supposed to have sex.

It's very high-stakes sex, and I'm amped up on hormones because of the Clomid, so "timed intercourse" is about as sexy as a transvaginal pelvic ultrasound. We get through it, then we wait a few weeks and return to the clinic for a pregnancy test. The test is negative. All that testing and all that monitoring and all that lack of privacy, and the cycle didn't even work.

FREQUENTLY ASKED QUESTION

I'm afraid of infertility treatments because I don't want to be the next Octomom. What happens if I end up with eight babies?

ANSWER: YOU HAVE WORSE THINGS TO WORRY ABOUT

Women going through infertility treatments are more likely to end up with multiples. Usually, this means twins or triplets. It could happen because you take a drug like Clomid, and when you ovulate, you produce two eggs. Then both eggs fertilize, and one of those fertilized embryos splits. Alternatively, you could be doing an IVF cycle where two embryos are transferred to your uterus and one splits. Or, theoretically, in either of those cases, you could have both embryos split, and that could give you four babies at once.

But I can tell you that there is a solid way to reduce your chances of having eight babies in one go. Just go to a reputable clinic, and if they tell you not to have sex at some particular time, don't have sex. I promise you, your risk of never having children is much higher than your risk of having eight children at once if you just listen to your doctor.

Any reputable fertility clinic will be monitoring the number of eggs you produce for a timed intercourse or Intra-uterine Insemination (IUI) cycle (more on what that is in a moment), and they will only transfer one or two embryos for an IVF cycle. If it looks like you've produced too many eggs or you are somehow ovulating during your IVF cycle, they will probably cancel the cycle or tell you not to have sex.

Problem avoided.[17]

By the way, don't hope for multiples, okay? Multiples are a blessing because all babies are blessings. Still, a multiples pregnancy is higher risk than a singleton (one baby) pregnancy. Twins and triplets are more likely than singletons to be born preemies or to be born with health complications.[18] I know it sounds wonderful to walk away from a cycle with twins and be able to end your infertility treatments in one go, but pay attention when the doctors tell you it's not something they suggest. (Or make friends with someone who has triplets. That mom loves her three kids like crazy. She can also give you the best lecture *ever* about why one baby at a time is best. Trust her.)

In any case, though, your worries of becoming Octomom are probably unfounded.

The realistic worry that you may not have thought about—and that you should think about now—is, "How am I going to keep feeling like a human as all these very intimate, private details about my life and body are revealed to dozens and dozens of people?"

And let's start answering this by talking about two of the easier types of infertility cycles a doctor can start you on. One is the scenario I described as my first treatment at the beginning of this chapter. It is referred to as a "timed intercourse" cycle, though I think they could relabel it "Drugs and Sex."[19]

With timed intercourse, your cycle begins when your next period starts, as always. Your fertility clinic then uses bloodwork and transvaginal pelvic ultrasounds to monitor the lining of your uterus, your ovaries, and your hormones. Based on what they see at the start of your cycle, they give you a drug like Clomiphene Citrate (Clomid) or Letrozole (Femara) to make you ovulate. They are careful with how much they prescribe because the clinic wants you to produce a couple of eggs, not a dozen.

In the meanwhile, you buy an ovulation kit from the drugstore. This is a set of sticks you pee on daily, much like a pregnancy test. The lines that show up on the sticks show you if you're about to ovulate. As you start to take your drugs, the clinic brings you in for monitoring appointments to check the eggs you're supposed to be growing in your ovaries like you're a chicken.

At some point, the ovulation kit and/or fertility clinic will tell you that you're about to ovulate. Then the clinic will tell you exactly when to have sex and how many times. (Or, if you have grown too many eggs, they may tell you not to have sex.) But assuming you have the number of eggs they want you to have and you're told to have sex, you and your partner will then have that prescribed timed intercourse.

After, you'll sit back and wait about ten days for a pregnancy test that you'll probably take at your clinic. This pregnancy test will be a blood test, and it's the earliest, most accurate way for your clinic to know if you're pregnant. You go to the clinic the morning of the test. They draw your blood. You chew your nails all day, and then a nurse or doctor calls you in the afternoon to tell you if you're pregnant.

Easy. Relatively.

Now, if Drugs and Sex don't get you pregnant, there are many steps up from there. My husband and I moved on from Drugs and Sex after our first cycle to Intrauterine Insemination (IUI), which you could call "Drugs and a Fancy Turkey Baster."[20]

For us, moving on to IUI meant after our first failed timed intercourse cycle, and as soon as my next period started, we went right back to the clinic. (A quick note here: ovulation triggers periods for me, so my "no periods" problem is temporarily resolved if I've just gone through an infertility cycle and it caused me to ovulate.)

The IUI cycle then began with another baseline appointment. I started taking Clomid. I went to the same monitoring appointments as I had before. But this time, they used what is called a "trigger shot" to force my body to ovulate when it looked like I had a ripe egg or two. They also collected sperm from my husband for the cycle, washed it (yep—that's a thing), and prepared it for IUI.

A day or so after the trigger shot, we went to the clinic, and the actual intrauterine insemination (sometimes called artificial insemination) was performed. To do this, the doctor threaded a tube up my cervix and injected my husband's washed sperm through that tube into my uterus. For me, this felt about the same as a saline ultrasound. From there, the sperm were supposed to swim through my fallopian tubes and find a ripe egg. After the procedure, we went home and waited those ten days again for the pregnancy test.

We tried IUI twice. It never worked. Still, timed inter-course and IUI were very good entry points for us, in the sense that they warmed us up to the indignities of infertility. When people who Don't Know talk about infertility, they tend to focus on physical discomfort and pain as the hard part of this. They imagine the horror of being on all those hormones and how painful it must be to have things stuck up and into your body all the time.

There *are* painful things about infertility—some of those diagnostic tests, the shots you later have to endure if you go through IVF—but the vast majority of the infertility proce-dures I've gone through were not that painful. They weren't pleasant. The hormones don't always make you feel *goo*. But it's not pain that makes infertility treatments start to feel like some kind of surreal nightmare you keep living over and over again. That comes from all the waiting we discussed in the last chapter and from repeatedly splaying yourself out for everyone to see while you try to engage in something that is meant to be an intimate process.

Let's compare to what a "normal" couple goes through

again. For most couples who are being proactive about family planning, the decision to "start trying" is a decision the two partners in the couple make together and without any outside help.

Maybe they chat about it over dinner for several weeks, then she goes off birth control and they stop buying condoms. They start having sex without anything to prevent pregnancy, and the first few times, that sex is epic, but very small scale. The couple is alone, maybe in their bedroom, possibly in their own bed. They might have the lights dimmed and the shades drawn. It's an act of love. They're doing something to make a life together. There's something sacred about it. The sex feels good. The couple feels closer after. This is how reproduction is supposed to work.

Now, take a couple going through IUI. Before that cycle starts, an entire fertility clinic is "in" on the couple's decision to try to get pregnant. The couple discusses what will happen with a doctor, then the woman must report to a nurse when her period starts and her cycle begins. After that, the woman will endure multiple appointments where she sits on an exam table, all "Winnie-the-Pooh," and someone other than her partner (who may or may not be present at those monitoring appointments) tells her to spread her knees apart and uses their hands and a wand with a condom on it to probe the woman.

In my experience, one cycle like that can involve three or four pelvic ultrasounds, and you might see a different doctor or nurse practitioner each time. There's often someone else in the room, too, like a nurse or tech, taking notes while the doctor or nurse practitioner does the ultrasound. If your partner is there, that's three people in the room who are watching as someone puts something up inside you. I've also had appointments like that where a nurse opens the exam room door from the outside and pops their head in to ask the doctor some urgent question during the ultrasound.

If you've never had a pelvic ultrasound, that might sound incredibly creepy. It's not so much. These are medical professionals. No one is staring at your vagina. No one is acting like it's fascinating to see that wand pushed up you. There's no plunging involve. The paper sheet is covering some things, and the doctor is in front of you, so there's not much of a view for anyone else. But you're still there, exposed, and a part of you that you were always told was "private" is very "public" for these appointments.

Your partner is going through this, too, by the way. He is usually sitting up near your head during the appointment. So while the nurse and doctor can see what the doctor is doing, your partner really can't. He's just watching the ultrasound on the video screen, same as you. And he is watching you—someone he presumably cares intimately about—while a bunch of other people get all up in the space that only he expected to be up in.

Your partner also has to go through his own embarrassment with this. Because his sperm has to be collected, and that means he either has to take home a kit to collect the sperm on his own, which he will then bring chilled to the clinic, or he has to show up at the clinic, go into a little room, and masturbate into a cup. If you think giving a urine sample sucks, you should try having to give a semen sample.

My husband had to do this several times. The first time, I went with him to the appointment and into the collection room. The room was tiny, and it had one chair I couldn't imagine anyone wanting to sit on, a sink, and some cupboards with dirty magazines and a few softcore porn videos. I do not exactly remember what went on during that "collection," which probably means it felt so degrading that I blocked the memory out later. He went on his own for the other "collections." I think it was easier for both of us to pretend it never happened if I wasn't there.

Finally, with that nasty exercise over and all your monitoring appointments finished, you and your partner get to the main event. The insemination. The part where the doctor actually puts your partner's sperm back inside you. Recall that the couple doing this the "old-fashioned" way is in a private space of their own. Probably, no one is watching. Probably, no one else even knows it's happening. That's not true for the couple doing this as an infertility exercise. For them, at least two other people are in the room, not just watching but actively involved.

For me, it was always difficult to be in that room and not think about how someone else was facilitating the transfer of my husband's sperm into my body. It never felt epic or sacred. It didn't feel special or romantic. It only ever felt clinical and kind of cold. I would be anxious walking out and worried it might not have worked. If I talked on the drive home, it would be nervous rambling.

I've asked my husband how he felt about that part of the cycle, and he had a more positive perspective. He said he felt hopeful. Which maybe goes to show some personality or gender difference. It's not that I *wasn't* hopeful after those procedures. It's that IUI represented such a loss of my own personal space that I dealt with it by disassociating a little. The alternative to letting it feel cold and clinical was to let it feel humiliating, awkward, uncomfortable, and degrading. "Hope" was something I could feel at home, but while I was spread wide for the world to see during those early cycles, letting a stranger help me and my husband get pregnant, the best I could manage was "holding still."

It was several years of infertility treatments before I realized that walking into a fertility clinic had become a true personal nightmare for me. I would enter the clinic—and it didn't matter which office or which clinic—and my eyes would register dull green furniture, dismal gray walls, and dirty yellow light. I would feel a light sense of vertigo as I smiled at the receptionist checking me in.

I would sit down in the waiting room, pull out my phone, and try not to feel sad about the other women and couples waiting there, too. If I was at a clinic where parents were allowed to bring children, and someone brought a child, I would try not to feel enraged. Then, when I was called back for my appointment, I would have the sensation that I was moving too fast while the world was moving too slow around me.

I was irritable with nurses, especially in later years, when I knew their routine better than they did. If they over-explained something, I perceived it as patronizing and got annoyed. I once snapped at a nurse who was trying to train a new staff member. She was talking me through what would happen at the pelvic ultrasound as if I hadn't been through dozens and dozens of these.

"This is my *sixth* IVF cycle," I said. "I know what to do." I resisted adding, "And maybe while you're training the new girl, you could advise her to look at her patient's chart before she starts talking to the patient. Because the women coming in here aren't exactly stress-free."

I told my therapist about the event later and confessed that I was still annoyed but also a little guilty. Those nurses hadn't meant to irritate me. No one ever means to make a woman with infertility feel worse. But at some point, the recurring nightmare sensation became so surreal and so depressing that I became a little snarky about it all. Or maybe hysterical is the right word. My husband, who lost some of his more naïve hope over the years and had to acquire a more patient hope, became much the same, and this eventually aged into some shared gallows humor.

But along with that humor came a certain sense of relief, and recently, I've noticed that not all the lights are yellow and not all the furniture is green. During my last appointments, I don't recall feeling myself disintegrating into the exam table. I also worry a lot less now about whether I'm perfectly shaved, bleeding a little, or whatever. I figure if you don't want to see what a real woman's vagina looks like, you shouldn't work at a fertility clinic.

I don't think the change has anything to do with my attitude being more positive, though. It's more that my perception of where dignity comes from has shifted. I used to think dignity had something to do with control over your own body, and maybe that was some remnant of my cultural upbringing. A dignified person bathes regularly, wears deodorant, and doesn't smell. A respectable person covers up the parts of herself that convey sexuality. A lady doesn't allow others to see hair on her legs or to know when she is on her period.

I couldn't keep any of that up with infertility, though. When you need help getting pregnant, strangers are going to see you vulnerable in the most intimate way. It's going to happen over and over again. Sometimes, it will hurt or feel uncomfortable. In response, your body could clench up. You could sweat. You could cry. You could bleed. Whatever happens, you won't be able to control much of it, nor will you be able to control who's watching.

So if "dignity" is about controlling your body and who sees it, then infertility is the epitome of indignity, and at some point, when you're going through that, you either have to stop yourself from feeling or you have to change how you think about dignity.

For me, it's helpful to redefine dignity for myself. Now, I think of dignity as the act of controlling my thoughts, not my body. When I am lying on that exam table, I do not choose to think about how making a life was supposed to be sacred and special and I'm stuck getting clinical and cold instead. I choose to tell myself that even though I didn't get that sacred, special experience, I did get something that proves I'm strong and capable of withstanding difficult things. When I think that way, I feel powerful instead of vulnerable, which somehow, cancels out the feeling that I'm losing dignity of any kind.

I don't know if there's a psychological term for that trick of the mind, but I have found that it is extremely good for me to re-frame my thoughts around ideas like dignity, privacy, vulnerability, power, and so on. I think this is another one of those hidden benefits of infertility. Turns out that if you can feel good about yourself while a probe is stuck up your vagina, a lot of things that might have otherwise embarrassed you or made you feel ashamed get easier. Conquer the pelvic ultrasound, and you can conquer all things. I swear it's true.

INFERTILITY LESSON #5

It is not easy to hand your body over to strangers, but if you can't get pregnant and you want babies that come out of your body, that's what you need to do. At first, that probably won't make you feel very good, but you can get through it. If I could go back in time and give myself some advice about *how*, it would be this:

1. Give yourself some grace. When your only experience with this kind of invasion is a run-of-the-mill pap smear, a transvaginal pelvic ultrasound could be a bad surprise. Multiple pelvic ultrasounds, over and over, will be a far cry from normal. If the privacy invasions of infertility don't feel good for you initially, give yourself permission to feel bad. You can't face feelings you stuff down and try to hide from. This isn't fun. It's okay to know that.

2. Challenge your own thoughts. If you're still having difficulty adjusting to that lack of privacy after a few cycles, start trying to challenge your own thoughts about what you're going through.

For example, suppose you hear yourself think, "This was supposed to be between my husband and me, and instead, it's between me, my husband, and a dozen fertility specialists." At that moment, try reminding yourself that those fertility specialists are helping you achieve a dream. Without their involvement, you might never have children. And it's not like you're having sex with everyone at the fertility clinic. You aren't!

3. Examine your feelings and beliefs. If you get to the point where trips to the fertility clinic feel like walking nightmares, try to figure out if you are holding on to feelings and beliefs you need to let go.

For example, do you feel "cold and clinical" at your appointments? If so, notice that, maybe observe those feelings for a while, and ask yourself why you feel that way. Is it because you believe procreation is supposed to be "sacred and warm?" Is it because the professionals in the room with you are, you know, so incredibly professional? Or is the room just really unpleasantly cold?

If your feelings stem from you focusing on the negatives of infertility, see if you can focus on the positives instead. Fix your mind on the possibilities you are creating, not what is technically happening to your body. Yes, there's a clinical professional injecting sperm into your uterus. But also, that medical intervention means you could be pregnant next week! There's hope behind what you're doing! This could be the time that works!

Alternatively, see if you need to replace an old belief with something new. If you believe conception is supposed to be a warm and sacred moment, and the cold clinic is violating this belief, maybe you need to shift that belief. Could conception be creative and hopeful instead? Because you can be those two things and cold at the same time.

Specifically with regard to dignity, if you, like me, at some point believed dignity was about control over your physical body, it's definitely time to change that belief. It was a false belief anyway. You never had as much control over your body as you thought. If you don't think that's true, ask someone older than you who's gone through some medical stress.

You do have control over the thoughts you let in, though. So when you're Donald Duck on an exam table, don't think of your exposed bottom. Think about how you are doing something other people fear. Think about your strength and endurance. Think of these things repeatedly, and when you walk out, tell yourself you could do what you just did a hundred times. You're just that good. You're just that unbreakable.

There's a heap of dignity in being able to withstand rough waters. Don't let yourself forget that.

FINAL THOUGHTS ON DIGNITY

There are so many misconceptions about infertility. The whole "what if I end up like Octomom" thing is probably the most laughable. It is far more serious and realistic to worry about how you're going to hold up to the emotional challenges infertility can bring.

Your ability to hand your body over to other people while still retaining your sense of who you are is important. This could go on for a while. You don't want to have to do it with the feeling that you're living in your own personal hell until it's over. The earlier you start taking back how this makes you feel, the better.

So suck it up, buttercup, and learn how not to give a damn if infertility forces you to lie back and spread yourself out for the world to see. Change your thoughts, give yourself something to feel good about, and revise your core beliefs if necessary.

If you can snort at a wand covered with a condom and some jelly and think, "You poorly designed dildo, I have defeated you!" then you can do just about anything. Plus, your capacity to tell dirty jokes will increase exponentially, and I'm pretty sure that particular skill is linked to longevity.[21]

CHAPTER SIX
Eggs Over Easy (Egg Retrieval)

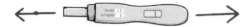

I'M AN EGG FACTORY

It is fall of 2014, and we have now completed one "timed intercourse" cycle (April) and two IUI cycles (May and June). We took off late summer and early fall because I was traveling for work too much to do another cycle then, and we needed a break. So far, we've spent about $6,871 on consults, diagnostic testing, the three cycles with all their monitoring and procedures, fertility drugs, and pregnancy tests.

This is what happens when your insurance does not cover infertility treatments. Frustratingly, we signed up for an insurance plan in 2014 that said it *did* cover fertility. Turns out, you need to read the fine print with insurance plans. Our insurance plan covered diagnostic testing for fertility problems, but it did not cover infertility *treatment*. The saline ultrasound and the HSG were covered but not the artificial insemination.

Also, since we had a high deductible plan, it didn't matter

practically that the diagnostic tests were technically "covered." It would have taken thousands of dollars for us to meet our out-of-pocket limit, and it took several thousand just to meet our deductible. Point being: we've paid for everything so far.

From here, we could keep trying with Clomid and IUI. After all, the Clomid does make me ovulate, and failure to ovulate is the only cause anyone can identify for our infertility. I just turned thirty-three, so age shouldn't be the issue. Presumably, we're simply not getting pregnant because no lucky sperm ever finds his way to an egg. Every IUI cycle costs about $2,200. Maybe we should put another $2,200 down on the table and press our bad luck.

Our doctor, however, is concerned that if these three cycles haven't done the trick, another won't do it, either. We are discouraged—emotionally, physically, and financially. I am eager to move on to something that might give us a better chance. Malcolm wants to limit the number of times I have to take super hormone drugs to get pregnant. In vitro fertilization (IVF) sounds like a faster guarantee. At least with IVF, we will know for sure that a fertilized egg made it to my uterus.[22] In January 2015, we start what is called a "fresh" IVF cycle.

IVF is more complicated than anything we've done before. First, the doctor recommends another saline ultrasound and that painful hysteroscopy I described in Chapter Four. We can't get these scheduled until January of 2015. Since the calendar year starts over then, doing these tests in January means we have to pay out-of-pocket for them. By January 12, we have paid the clinic another $3,142, and we haven't even gotten to the costs of IVF itself.

When the tests show that we're ready to move forward,

we plunk down $13,125 out-of-pocket for the IVF cycle itself. We are paying for the baseline appointment, monitoring appointments, egg retrieval and sperm collection, fertilization of the eggs, and the embryo transfer itself. Our payment does not include the medications or the pregnancy test at the end of the cycle. The pregnancy test is at least covered by insurance, though. It only costs $25.

At the time, I do not look closely at the total amount of money we are spending. It has started to feel too stressful to look at that financial bleed all at once, so we focus on one payment at a time and know we are extremely lucky and blessed to be able to afford this. These costs would be prohibitive for many couples.

I start the IVF cycle similarly to how I start most cycles. I take birth control for two weeks, stop the birth control, call the nurse when my period starts, and go to the clinic for a baseline appointment. The baseline is the same as it was for the IUI cycles: transvaginal pelvic ultrasound plus bloodwork. The nurse calls me in the afternoon to tell me my estrogen levels are low (that's how they should be), and I get the go-ahead to start my injections three days later.

The purpose of the injections is to stimulate my ovaries, and a specialty fertility pharmacy ships the meds and supplies to my front door in an insulated box. The box contains vials of medication, piles of syringes, alcohol swabs, and a big red sharps container.

Malcolm and I watch a video to learn how to do the injections, and he tries to do the injection for me the first night. This is the first time he's had to do something like this, though, and he's afraid of hurting me, so he pushes the needle in too slow and with slightly shaking hands.

Those needles are sharp. What I need him to do is jab

me with that needle, like it's a dart. These are tummy shots. If he jabs fast, the needle will slide into my stomach fat like a hot knife through butter. By doing it slow and trying to avoid hurting me, he's inadvertently jiggling an extremely sharp instrument around inside me.

I fire him from his job. I am perfectly capable of pinching my belly fat and jabbing myself fast with a needle, and actually, this turns out to be the least difficult part of the whole cycle. The needle is sharp, and it looks kind of long, but it's extremely thin. I hardly feel it at all.

Well, that's not entirely honest. I don't feel it for the first few days. After that, my stomach starts to bruise, and that's when those needles start to hurt. Turns out that jabbing a bruise always hurts, no matter how fast you do it. After a week of shots, my stomach is black and blue and sore.

Still, I feel that the hype about IVF injections is just hype. The injections aren't the bad part about this. The bad part is the way the drugs make me feel. I do not mean "feel" in the emotional sense. Yes, I'm a little irritable from the massive amount of hormones I'm taking, but now I'm feeling internal physical discomfort, too. The injections make my ovaries produce far more eggs than they would normally make in a cycle, and I turn out to be a super-responder. My ovaries produce tons of eggs in response to those drugs, and my belly becomes bloated and achy while it happens.

A "fresh" IVF cycle involves two main parts. The first part is ovarian stimulation, followed by an egg retrieval procedure. The second is egg fertilization, followed by an embryo transfer procedure.[23] The procedures occur about a week apart. Right now, we're focused on ovarian stimulation and egg retrieval. I take about twelve days of injections, and I need monitoring appointments at the clinic every other day or so after the seventh day. This is serious egg checking, and I feel like a chicken again. By the time the doctor decides my eggs are ready, my ovaries are over-worked, my estrogen levels are sky-high, my belly is huge, and I'm constipated, irritable, and tired (thank you, hormones).

Finally, the day of the egg retrieval arrives. The egg retrieval takes place at the fertility clinic in a special area set up for surgical procedures. During the procedure, the doctor uses various instruments to go in through your vagina and up to your ovaries to collect the eggs. My layman's understanding is that the collection is basically the doctor vacuuming eggs from your ovaries, but I didn't go to medical school. Probably it's far more complicated than that. For my purposes, what matters is it's a vaginal surgery, and I'm not going to be awake for it.

Malcolm and I go together to a little pre-op room before the procedure. A nurse hands me a robe ("it opens in the back"), a cloth sheet ("for you to wrap around your waist until we get in the room"), thick blue socks with plastic grips on the soles, and a hair net. Everything else I'm wearing comes off. Then we sit in the pre-op room while the nurse goes over various information and asks me questions about whether I've been fasting, what I'm allergic to, etc.

The nurse starts an IV. I am thankful to have large, juicy veins again, but even I dislike IVs. There's just something about someone inserting a tube into my blood vessels that bothers me. Also, I don't like how IVs sting my skin. Still, it's a minor annoyance because at least they don't have any trouble sticking me. I am a little dehydrated because I've been fasting, but the nurse starts a saline drip through the IV, and I feel that hydration almost immediately. That, at least, is a positive.

An anesthesiologist comes to talk to me, and I think the anesthesiologist is very attractive. I learn over the years that I *always* think this about anesthesiologists, regardless of whether they are old, young, male, female. I'd probably think a sea monster working as an anesthesiologist was attractive. There's just something about a doctor who can take the pain away that makes that person inherently and wildly good looking. In my humble opinion, anesthesiologists are gods disguised as humans.

Soon after I speak to the anesthesiologist, the nurse walks me to the operating room, and two nurses help me onto a table with enormous stirrups This is the scariest part of the egg retrieval, and later, I think it's the icky part of any vaginal surgery.

There are multiple people in the room with you, and you're meeting most of them for the first time while you're barely clothed. These people help you position your bottom at the edge of a table and put your calves up into those stirrups, which force you to spread your legs open enough so there's plenty of room for a doctor to get between your knees. You're in an incredibly vulnerable position by the time they have you ready for the surgery.

This egg retrieval is my first time going through something like this, and I'm anxious. But then, the *rugs*. Oh, the drugs! I have never done any street drugs in my life. Never smoked marijuana. Tried a cigar once in my late twenties and was completely grossed out. Probably that's a very good thing, because I'm a big fan of drugs that put you out for surgeries.

Thanks to those drugs, I hardly remember what goes on after my legs are in the stirrups. Someone puts a warm blanket over my chest. Someone says they've started the anesthesia. A light buzz washes over me, and just like that, I'm off in a dream world where I feel no trouble whatsoever about anything.

When I wake up, I'm in a recovery area, and Malcolm is sitting nearby. It takes a minute or so for the groggy feeling to start wearing off. I don't feel any significant pain. The nurse gives me graham crackers and juice. The doctor comes around to tell me I did great. They collected thirty-six eggs. Of those, six had to be discarded, but thirty were high enough quality to fertilize. That's so many that they had to decide what to do with them all! The doctor explains that they split the batch in half. They're going to try to fertilize twelve, and they'll freeze the other eighteen.

"Because we don't want to put all your eggs in one basket," is what he says. I think. I might have made that up in my mind as the drugs were wearing off. But that's the basic message. I don't question it. Seems like a good idea to me.

I go home, take some pain meds, and spend the rest of the afternoon sleeping. It takes a few days for the bloat to wear off, but I have a medication to help with that, and I drink a lot of water. I don't realize until much later that lots of women don't need that medication. I'm hyperstimulated, though, and that can cause dangerous bloating if you don't stay hydrated after.[24]

Now that the egg retrieval is over, we're on to the second part of the cycle: egg fertilization and embryo transfer. I do not need the ovarian stimulation meds anymore, but two days after the retrieval, I have to start progesterone shots.

Unfortunately, Malcolm does have to do these for me because the needles are bigger, the oil the progesterone sits in is too thick to inject quickly, and you have to take those shots in the rear. Once he gets used to stabbing me with the needles, they don't hurt any worse than the stomach shots, but Malcolm always drinks a glass of wine before he does the shot every night. To make it easier for him.

Pretty sure this is when I decide that women are significantly stronger than men. *He* needs something to relax so that he can give *me* an injection? Where's my glass of wine!? I just have to suck it up and deal.

(Sweetheart, I love you, but you would never have survived what I have survived.)

This is an exciting time, though, because we're also getting updates about what's going on with the egg fertilization. The embryologist, a fertility specialist who creates those embryos from the eggs retrieved and sperm collected during an IVF cycle, calls us every day or so after the retrieval for the next five days. For seven of the twelve eggs, the lab basically accomplishes fertilization by mixing sperm with egg in a petri dish. For the other five, the lab uses Intracytoplasmic Sperm Injection (ICSI) to fertilize the eggs. ICSI is a process where one sperm is injected into one egg, and it is supposed to give you a greater chance of any egg fertilizing successfully.[25]

Of the five eggs injected by ICSI, four successfully fertilize. Of the seven mixed in the dish, five successfully fertilize. So that's nine fertilized eggs, and five days after the fertilization, one of those fertilized eggs is now an embryo that is high enough quality for our embryo transfer.

We go in for the procedure that day, and the embryo transfer is much easier than the egg retrieval. We start in the same pre-op room, and I am given the same "outfit" I was given for the egg retrieval. However, this time I get to keep my bra on, and no IV is needed because I'll be awake. Malcolm also gets accessories—shoe covers and a hair net—since he gets to be in the room for the transfer.

I have to arrive with a full bladder because the doctor needs your bladder full for an embryo transfer so that they can see on an ultrasound where exactly they're putting the embryo. My bladder fills fast, and it seems like an awfully long time between when we arrive and when they finally take us back from the pre-op room to the procedure room. Then I have to lay on a table and put my feet up in stirrups again while the nurse presses down on my stomach with an ultrasound wand to see if my bladder is full enough.

It's full enough. I'm having a hard time holding it. Thankfully, the procedure gets underway fast. The embryologist brings us a picture of the embryo—"Look! It's already hatching!"—and the doctor comes into the room.

The doctor threads a catheter up through my cervix and does a "practice" run to make sure there is a clear path to my uterus. The embryologist brings in the embryo itself. We get a picture of the embryo—our first picture of the baby! Then we watch on a monitor while the doctor inserts the embryo into my uterus. The actual procedure only takes about ten minutes. I finally get to pee! Malcolm and I walk out feeling extremely hopeful.

We get a call from the embryologist the next day, and we learn that two more of the fertilized eggs are embryos that are high enough quality for IVF. These "Day Six" embryos are frozen for future cycles. The lab discards the remaining fertilized eggs because they either aren't big enough or the cells aren't dividing or they are "arresting" (read: dying) already.

Ten days after the transfer, I return to the clinic for a pregnancy test, and I'm pregnant! A month after that, I'm not. But that's another part of my story.

FREQUENTLY ASKED QUESTION

I'm in my late twenties or early thirties, and I'm ultra-focused on my career right now. I'm not married yet, and I do want kids, but not for years. Should I freeze my eggs?

ANSWER: FREEZING YOUR EGGS IS HARD

On television, when a young woman goes to a fertility clinic to freeze her eggs, it is a process that seems to happen magically and all in one or two appointments. The young woman walks into the clinic, sits awkwardly in the waiting room, and walks out with a pamphlet of information. She tells her best friend or her boyfriend a few scenes later that she's freezing her eggs. Those eggs are collected and frozen before the episode ends.

In magazine and news articles, when "freezing your eggs" comes up, it is normally in the context of advice to career women. Watch out! Your eggs are only good for so long! You might be running out! If you want to wait until you're thirty-five to have kids, you better freeze those eggs now! Run off to a clinic and make that happen. It would be irresponsible not to.

Now look, it is true that women have a limited number of eggs and younger eggs are more easily fertilized than older eggs.[26] So, if you have the time, energy, and money to get your eggs frozen when you're in your late twenties, I say, go for it! Freeze those eggs. You might be very happy to have done it later.

That being said, I think the pressure put on young women

to worry about their eggs to the point of freezing them is extremely ill-informed. Because what the media *never* tells you is that freezing your eggs is an intense, expensive, and time-consuming process.

Freezing your eggs doesn't mean just going to a clinic at the right time in your cycle and letting your doctor scrape a few eggs from your ovaries. Egg retrieval involves multiple appointments and potent drugs that overwork your ovaries so there will be more than one egg to collect.

It is only very rarely covered by insurance, and if you have to pay out-of-pocket, it can cost thousands of dollars. In total, our first IVF cycle, including the consult, the tests, the drugs, the monitoring, the procedures, the pregnancy test, and the D&C I had after I miscarried, cost about $17,407. The egg retrieval is only half of a fresh IVF cycle, so it probably wouldn't cost as much for just that part, but it would be reasonable to budget $10,000 for an egg retrieval.[27] That's a pretty high expense for a young woman.

Additionally, egg retrieval takes far more than one appointment. You'll have to go in for a consult, a baseline appointment, monitoring, and the egg retrieval itself. You won't be able to schedule most of those appointments at your convenience because once your cycle starts, your body will decide for you how long it takes to produce ripe eggs.

I would recommend expecting four-to-six weeks to pass from the initial consult to your egg retrieval, but it could take much longer, depending on your fertility clinic's schedule. Also, the injections don't usually take more than two weeks, but while you're on them, you'll feel—at best—irritable and bloated. At worst, you will face hyperstimulation, which can be dangerous and life-threatening.[28] (I got irritable, bloated, and hyperstimulated, but thankfully not to the life-threatening extent. It was still a lousy feeling.)

The day of the retrieval, you will need someone else to come with you because you will be put under for the procedure. When you wake up, you could learn that they were able to collect 40 eggs, or you could learn that they were only able to collect 4. Either way, you won't be working that day. You'll be resting. Expect to take the day off. You'll need it. You're going to work hard for those eggs.

INFERTILITY LESSON #6

So you want to "focus on your career" and wait to have kids until you're thirty-six? Then my very non-medical opinion[29] is that yes, you should freeze your eggs. Don't expect it to be easy. It won't be. You will spend a lot of time, money, and energy on this. But if you *have* lots of time, money, and energy to spare, why not?

Also, I'm *sure* the average woman in her late twenties has *plenty* of work flexibility and absolutely nothing to spend $10,000 on other than freezing her eggs.

(She said, snarkily.)

If you decide that you *don't* have the resources to freeze your eggs, try to forgive yourself. It's not a perfect world. Your life isn't a television drama. All you can do is the best you can do, and egg freezing is a luxury item.

In an ideal world, you would get to grow your career when you need to, "lean in," and then pull those eggs out of the freezer to thaw when you have time for kids in your late thirties. But since it's not an ideal world, most career women who also want kids will have to make some hard choices about family planning.

It's impossible to know how this will all play out for you ten years from now, whether you freeze your eggs or not. It's impossible to know what you will and won't regret. **Make the best choice you can with your eggs, and don't let some expert—or your mom—scare you too much. You can only do what you can do.**

A "FRESH" IVF CYCLE

Now, for most readers, I'm guessing egg retrieval will be most relevant to you as part of the IVF process. So for you, egg retrieval will be one half of a fresh IVF cycle.

By the way, in case this wasn't clear from my story, a fresh IVF cycle is when they use recently collected sperm to fertilize recently collected eggs, then cultivate whatever embryos result from that process for a few days (usually three or five) until a fresh embryo is available to be inserted back into the woman's body. Extra embryos get frozen for later tries (which are called "frozen" IVF cycles).[30]

A fresh IVF cycle is what most people think of when they talk about IVF, and it's kind of the "big leagues" of infertility treatments, at least in terms of time, costs, physical demand, etc. It will run you anywhere from $10,000 to $25,000. It may not be covered by insurance. It will take six-to-eight weeks to complete. You will be in the doctor's office all the time. You probably won't feel very good.

Oh, and it might not work. The Society for Assisted Reproductive Technology (SART) reports that in 2017 in the U.S., a woman aged 35 to 37 doing IVF only had a 31.6% chance of getting pregnant with her first embryo transfer from a fresh IVF cycle. The chances were only 40.5% for women younger than 35.[31] So your chance of getting pregnant with one fresh IVF cycle is probably about as high as your chance of winning a game of rock, paper, scissors.

A lot of IVF clinics offer "deals" where you spend a higher amount of money now, and in return you are guaranteed a baby after a certain number of cycles or you get your money back. Beware: those programs often come with limiting clauses. Like, you must complete X number of cycles in X number of years and not have a baby in that time to get your money back. You can't necessarily jump clinics. You may still have to pay for medications. Check the fine print and do the math before you sign up for an IVF deal.

Additionally, you should know that your fresh cycle could occur in two cycles, which could be separated by weeks, months, or even years. That could happen if you start with the ovarian stimulation, egg retrieval, and egg fertilization, then you freeze all your embryos.

Why would you do that? Genetic testing, probably. Your fertility lab can send tiny cell biopsies (samples) from your embryos off to a genetics company that can tell you whether your embryos are likely to have chromosomal abnormalities or certain specific genetic disorders. If you do genetic testing on all your embryos, you will schedule your frozen cycle later, likely with your best normal embryo.

Malcolm and I chose to go that route the second time we did an egg retrieval, partly because I produced so many eggs the first time and my body was so swollen after that we later wondered if that hurt our first little embryo's chances of success.

But speaking of those eggs we harvested the first time …

ARRESTED DEVELOPMENT

It is summer 2017, and we've completed three IVF cycles. That's our fresh cycle plus two frozen cycles. Now, we're out of embryos. Luckily, we have those eighteen eggs from our egg retrieval left on ice. That's six more than the number they fertilized the first time, so we assume we'll get a fair number of embryos out of this batch of eggs.

It turns out that fertilizing eggs isn't free, though. We have to pay for another sperm collection and pay for the egg fertilization, too. Then we wait. The embryologist calls us a day or so after the fertilization. Of those eighteen eggs, over half did not tolerate the thaw. Only eight fertilized and are being cultured.

I have a sickening feeling as I start frantically searching the Internet for information about whether eggs or embryos freeze better. I find a few random articles suggesting that eggs don't survive the freezing and thawing process as well as embryos. Some confirmation bias kicks in, and I immediately wonder why the fertility clinic decided to freeze any eggs if embryos have a better chance of surviving. Also, why are we paying for a second sperm collection and second fertilization process? We wouldn't have had to pay for this if they'd fertilized all the eggs at once, would we?

My paranoia increases when the embryologist calls me two days later. It's bad news. I can tell from the tone of her voice. Of the eight eggs that fertilized, only *two* have made it to the Day Five or Day Six embryo stage. The others "arrested." That means they died.

I am sitting in a parking lot in my car when I get that call, and I feel like I've had the wind knocked out of me.

Two embryos? We had eighteen eggs, and we only got *two* embryos!? That's hardly any chance for a pregnancy at all!

I cry because I am devastated and because I am furious. I do not understand why the fertility clinic chose this path. I feel that anger for a long time before it simmers down. Ultimately, I decide that the research on freezing eggs versus freezing embryos does not clearly show that one is better than the other. I think the clinic really did have our best interests in mind when they froze half the eggs.

At the same time, I never quite get over the fact that they made that decision for us. The opportunity to choose what happened with any extra eggs should have been ours. We might have made the same choice, but who knows? We should have been asked about this before the retrieval, too. It shouldn't have come up for the first time while I was still groggy from anesthesia.

Eighteen eggs.

Two embryos.

INFERTILITY LESSON #7

Before you go through with your retrieval, talk to your clinic about what they're going to do with the eggs. If they only harvest a few, they'll probably assume you want all eggs fertilized. But what happens if you get twenty eggs? Thirty? Forty?

Try to imagine many possible scenarios. I know women who only get a handful of eggs from any retrieval but have great success with the fertilization process. You can start with ten eggs and end up with three embryos of the highest grade. Or, you can start with thirty-six and end up with four low-grade embryos. You won't know in advance.

Do your research on the survival rates of frozen eggs as opposed to frozen embryos. And I don't just mean "Google it." When I wrote this, as a layperson writing a memoir about my personal experiences, I was unable to find recent research on how likely it is for a frozen egg versus a frozen embryo to survive the thawing process. I couldn't find the Internet articles I thought I'd read years ago that said embryos thaw better than eggs, either.

You may be able to find information I couldn't, but if you can't, you do have another research option. You can ask your clinic what their statistics are. Your fertility clinic may be able to tell you what percentage of frozen eggs survive the thawing process in their lab versus what percentage of frozen embryos survive.

Even if your clinic does not have those statistics, you can still ask your doctor what they recommend and make a plan with your partner. Importantly, do all of this before your egg retrieval, not immediately after, when the anesthesia may prevent you from thinking straight. There may not be a perfect decision, and you might not have all the information you want, but you can at least make the call when you're not on drugs!

Beware that there are other considerations with eggs and embryos. In particular, there are papers you will need to sign about what happens to your eggs and embryos if you and your partner divorce or if one or both of you die. Read those papers and make that decision carefully. Keep in mind that infertility is tough on love.

Finally, if you're planning a fresh IVF cycle, get information about your costs before you begin, not just for this cycle but for future frozen cycles and fertilizations. Plan for weeks of drugs and monitoring appointments, and make sure you don't have a vacation or business trip that will conflict. A little forethought will go a long way here.

FINAL THOUGHTS ON EGGS

Egg retrieval is intense. A fresh IVF cycle is even more intense. This will probably be the most physically difficult part of your infertility journey if you have to do it. Take care of yourself during this time. You will see later that for me, that first fresh IVF cycle and the miscarriage that followed threw me into a tailspin from which I needed two years to recover. This will be easier on you if you are physically and emotionally healthy before you begin.

CHAPTER SEVEN
Test Tube Babies (IVF)

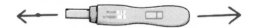

HELL IS FROZEN

It is spring of 2017. After our first fresh IVF cycle ended in miscarriage, we needed time to heal. But now, things are looking up. We decide it's time to get back on the horse, and we make an appointment at our fertility clinic. At this point, we are familiar with several of the doctors there. Although we feel we received good care from all the doctors, there is one we particularly like. We communicate easily with her, and her smart-but-laid-back style matches what we want in a doctor. We set up a consult with her to talk about IVF.

We have two embryos frozen right now from the fresh IVF cycle, so this time around, we can do a frozen IVF cycle.[32] Frozen cycles are less intense than fresh cycles, and they're less expensive even if you don't have insurance. And this time we do have insurance that covers IVF. It's a high-de-ductible plan, but we'll take what we can get.

I start a frozen cycle in May 2017. Because our insurance

is a high-deductible plan, we still have to pay an IVF "deposit" of $1,984 to cover what the clinic thinks our insurance won't cover. We also have to pay $251 for another saline ultrasound (because the testing never ends) and we haven't yet met our deductible. But sometime later in the year some of our costs will be covered!

I've been on birth control, but I stop the birth control and call the nurse when my period starts so I can go in for a baseline appointment. Same drill as always. Transvaginal pelvic ultrasound and bloodwork. By now, I'm used to this part of an infertility treatment cycle. The appointment is no big deal.

Everything is fine with my bloodwork, and I get a call from the nurse in the afternoon. She tells me to start taking estrogen pills. I head back for a monitoring appointment a week later, and then I'm ready to start progesterone shots. There are no stomach shots required for a frozen cycle because your ovaries aren't tasked with making any eggs during a cycle like this. The estrogen and progesterone together make me feel a little high-strung after a few days, but compared to what a fresh cycle requires in terms of hormones and medications, this is nothing.

On June 15, 2017, Malcolm and I go together to the clinic for our embryo transfer. This part is the same as it was for the fresh IVF cycle. I have a full bladder so they can see my uterus clearly with an ultrasound. I over-hydrated this time, though, and my bladder is so full I get told by the nurse to go empty some of it. She says, "Count to ten while you're peeing, then stop." Right ... I'll just do that with my super full bladder.

I do my best emptying only part of my bladder, then I return to the procedure room from the bathroom. I get situated on the table. The nurse puts a picture of my uterus back up on the monitor. The embryologist enters the room and shows us a picture of the unfrozen embryo.

The doctor comes in. She inserts a catheter through my cervix, does a "practice run" to make sure she has a clear path, then threads the embryo up into my uterus.

The whole event takes about an hour from check in to check out. The time between when Malcolm and I are taken back to the procedure room and when I am finally allowed to empty my bladder completely is only about ten minutes, maybe less. We go home and get back to work.

Whatever happens from here is all up to fate, luck, God, or whoever controls miracles. Our pregnancy test is scheduled for ten days from now, and I spend that whole time over-analyzing every cramp. Do my boobs hurt a little? Was that twinge I just felt the embryo implanting? There's no way to know. Pregnancy symptoms can be so similar to what you feel before your period comes that pretty much anything you feel during that wait is impossible to interpret.

I'm convinced it worked this time anyway. Things seem to have gone so smoothly. But it didn't work. The pregnancy test is negative. We try again with the second embryo in August, and again, it doesn't work. No pregnancy.

Something is wrong. The doctor suggests a "mock" embryo cycle with a uterine biopsy for Endometrial Receptivity Analysis (ERA), which is like an IVF cycle in terms of medications and shots. However, instead of ending with an embryo transfer, a mock embryo cycle for ERA ends with a doctor biopsying your uterus—which means snipping out part of your uterus—and sending that sample to a lab for analysis.[33]

The biopsy is incredibly painful and kind of bloody, and

you do it without anesthesia because it's too short for them to put you out for the procedure. Also, you have to do all the same estrogen and progesterone you would do for a real IVF cycle, even though the mock cycle never gives you a chance at getting pregnant. The goal of the biopsy and ERA is to determine if your body needs a little more or a little less progesterone during a real IVF cycle. It's a lot of work for an extra day or so of progesterone. Still, supposedly, this can make a significant difference in an IVF cycle.

After the mock cycle, we have the rest of our frozen eggs fertilized. This is what I described in the last chapter. We have eighteen frozen eggs, but we only get two embryos from those eggs.

We start a third frozen IVF cycle. Our clinic has a "one is best" policy, and we have only ever had the doctors insert one embryo during an embryo transfer. But we're batting zero, and I am thirty-five years old. We assume our chances of multiples are low, even if we transfer two embryos at once. We're also hemorrhaging money on infertility, and we suspect that we may have to do another fresh IVF cycle after this. We ask the clinic to transfer both of our remaining embryos during this frozen cycle.

The decision turns out not to matter. When the clinic thaws the two embryos for our embryo transfer, one of the embryos is already arresting. They transfer both embryos anyway in the hopes that one takes. Neither does. Our pregnancy test is negative. Again.

We take a break from IVF in winter of 2018 because we're tired, and we go back to timed intercourse for three cycles. Then in summer 2018, we make that move to North Carolina, get hooked up with a new fertility clinic and a new doctor, and start diagnostic testing and infertility treatments all over again. We do another egg retrieval, genetic testing, another mock embryo cycle, and two additional frozen IVF cycles between August 2018 and November 2019.

We get a negative pregnancy test on the first IVF cycle with the new clinic, then, finally, we get a positive on the next. That pregnancy ends in miscarriage.

That's two egg retrievals, one fresh embryo transfer, five frozen embryo transfers, seven embryos, and two mock cycles. Six chances to get pregnant, or seven if you count each embryo as a chance. Four negative pregnancy tests. Two positive pregnancy tests. Two pregnancies. Two miscarriages.

If you add in the four timed intercourse cycles we've gone through and the two IUI cycles, we're up to twelve chances to get pregnant, ten negative pregnancy tests, two positive pregnancy tests, two pregnancies, and two miscarriages.

In the years when I am doing all that, which run from 2014 to 2019, I also travel the world for a negotiation training and consulting company. I start a solo law practice, then a consulting firm with a partner, then a publishing business. I publish seven books under three names. Malcolm makes partner, then goes in-house as an attorney.

We make the move from Georgia (where we at least had an aunt and uncle that I'm close with and a community we cared about) to North Carolina (where we initially have no friends and no family whatsoever). I gain thirty pounds, lose twenty pounds, gain ten pounds, lose ten pounds, gain fifteen pounds, lose five pounds, basically all from stress eating, something which is much harder for me to control when my hormones are being hijacked by IVF cycles.

Those are hard years, and there are times when I'm bitter. There are times when someone says, "keep trying,"

and I want to hand my medical bills over and ask the igno-
rant person if they would like to pay these bills and take the
weight I've gained and put it on their thighs. There are also
times when I am stronger than that. There are times when I
move on and pursue dreams and set new, non-baby related
goals. But if I'm totally honest, even when I'm feeling strong,
I'm angry with God.

FREQUENTLY ASKED QUESTION

I just went through an egg retrieval and that was hell.
Now I'm gearing up for a frozen IVF cycle. Surely it can't get
worse? (Please tell me it doesn't get worse.)

ANSWER: THE ODDS ARE AGAINST YOU

Here's the good news about IVF: the fresh cycles are
the hard work. They're the serious drugs, the ovarian stimulation, the bloating, the procedure you have to do with
anesthesia, the stress over how many eggs will be collected
and how many of those will become good embryos, and
the embryo transfer and waiting to see if you're pregnant
on top of all that. The fresh IVF cycles are also the expensive cycles. Those are the ones where you're likely to spend
$15,000. Or more.

After you get your fresh cycle over with, though, you
might have a few leftover embryos that you can freeze. So
the next time you want to try IVF, you can use one of those
frozen embryos instead of needing to go back and do another
egg retrieval again.

A frozen IVF cycle (sometimes called a "FET" cycle for "frozen embryo transfer" cycle) is when they prepare your body for a pregnancy with estrogen and progesterone, then unfreeze an embryo and insert it into your uterus right around the time you would have conceived in a normal pregnancy.

Compared to a fresh cycle, a frozen cycle requires less drugs, takes less time, and costs less money. In my experience, frozen cycles run between $2,000 and $5,000. However, I've never been able to find any good research that would tell me the average cost of a frozen cycle in the U.S. I think this is because it's difficult to calculate an average cost for a frozen IVF cycle. Many frozen cycles depend on fresh cycles, because unless you are using donor embryos (which is basically you adopting an embryo that some other couple was willing to donate), you had to do a fresh cycle to get a frozen embryo in the first place. Also, some frozen cycles are baked into the cost of a fresh cycle. For these reasons, it would be hard to know what a typical frozen cycle costs.

But to answer the question this chapter asks: if you are looking side-by-side at one fresh IVF cycle and one frozen IVF cycle, the frozen cycle is far easier than the fresh cycle. So no, it doesn't get worse.

Except, it kind of does.

If you end up needing multiple frozen cycles, then over time, that series of frozen cycles can be much worse than one fresh cycle.

A lot of women don't need as many frozen cycles as I've needed, so this may not matter to you. For some women, the fresh cycle works the very first time, and no additional cycle is needed. For others, the fresh cycle might never produce eggs or embryos that are high enough quality to result in any pregnancy. In that case, they may never move on to frozen embryos. Then there are times when money is a factor. If you don't have good insurance and your wallet is stretched too thin, you might have embryos left after a fresh cycle but not be able to use them because you can't afford it.

If, however, you are in shoes like mine, and you end up having to do multiple frozen cycles, then at some point, the cumulative stress of all those cycles could become a hell far worse than the stress of one fresh IVF cycle. That's because even though the frozen cycles are easier, the fatigue of infertility really hits when you're on the third or fourth frozen cycle. That's when you find yourself deep in the circles of infertility hell, spent, exhausted, and nearly defeated.

Also, even if you're only on your first frozen IVF cycle, there's a certain torture that happens when any frozen cycle fails. It's just easy to feel that by the time you get to a frozen cycle, you've already had your fair share of failure. You assume the odds should be in your favor by now. So it's a real slap in the face each time a frozen cycle fails.

Unfortunately, the belief that the odds are *ever* on your side is a false belief. The odds are against you from the very beginning. Here are some statistics to consider:

1. Infertility is extremely common. According to the CDC, about 6% of married women aged 15 to 44 years in the United States can't get pregnant after one year of trying. About 12% of women (married or not) in the same age range in the U.S. have difficulty getting pregnant or carrying a pregnancy to term.[34]

2. A normal couple is more likely not to get pregnant than to get pregnant on any given cycle. Even on the day before you ovulate—the most fertile day of a woman's cycle—the overall chances of conceiving are only 42%.[35]

3. Age affects fertility. A woman's fertility gradually declines in her thirties, and things get ugly after age 35. On average, a thirty-year-old woman trying to get pregnant has a 20% chance in any cycle. For a forty-year-old woman, that number drops to only 5%.

Most women become unable to get pregnant sometime in their mid-40s, whether they are using infertility treatments or not, and this is because as you age, the quality and quantity of your eggs drop. (Men do not have the same problem. Sperm quality drops as men age, too, but it's not usually an issue before a guy reaches his 60s. There is not a maximum age at which a man stops being able to get a woman pregnant.)[36]

4. Your likelihood of success with IUI is about as high as your likelihood of success with natural conception. If you're under 35, you have a 10-20% chance of pregnancy with an IUI cycle. If you're between 35 and 40, you have about a 10% chance. If you're over 40, your chances are only 2-5%.[37]

5. Your likelihood of success with IVF depends on your age and may take multiple tries. The Society for Assisted Reproductive Technology (SART) reported the data in the table below on the percentages of live births (one baby) that resulted from egg retrieval cycles and embryo transfers in the U.S. in 2017.

Note that even for women younger than 35, the chance of having a baby from an egg retrieval, either from the first embryo transfer or subsequent embryo transfers, was only 54.7%. For women aged 38 to 40, that number was 25.6%.[38]

Go check these statistics out yourself at the SART website, which has all kinds of data and is likely to have more recent data by the time I hit "publish" on this memoir.

Woman's age	<35	35-37	38-40	41-42	>42
Chance of having a live birth from an egg retrieval and any subsequent embryo transfer	54.7%	40.6%	25.6%	12.8%	4.4%
Chance of having a live birth from an egg retrieval on your first embryo transfer	40.5%	31.6%	21.5%	11.2%	4.0%
Chance of having a live birth from second or later embryo transfer	45.9%	42.8%	38.5%	34.7%	28.6%

Generally, what I'm trying to get at here is that your chance of having a baby during any cycle, whether it's an infertility treatment cycle or not, is probably always worse than the chance of flipping "heads" on a coin toss. Roll the dice enough times with a 30% chance of rolling "baby," and you'll probably roll "baby" eventually. Still, the keyword there is "probably." These cycles are all independent of each other. Doing one doesn't prime your body for better odds the second time.

Also, you could be doing everything right and just get unlucky time and time again. Or there could be something wrong you don't know about. I thought for years that not ovulating was my big problem. Then in 2019, I learned that I also have a condition called adenomyosis, which is like endometriosis.[39] Both conditions affect the lining of your uterus and can make it harder to get pregnant.

So what exactly caused my infertility? Polycystic Ovarian Syndrome? Adenomyosis? Poor luck? We do not know. Could be all of the above. Could be none of the above. Certainly, the fact that I was at this for years didn't help. Your chances of success do not go up as you age.

By the way, it's not always the woman causing the problem. Sometimes it's the man. According to the CDC, in about 35% percent of cases, a male factor is identified along with a female factor. In 8%, a male factor is the only identifiable cause.[40]

Are there things you can do to improve your chances? Supposedly. Age, weight, alcohol and tobacco use, exercise, irregular periods, and STDs are all considered "risk factors" for infertility.[41] Since I'm not a doctor or medical professional of any kind, and this is all based on my personal experience and the research I've done on the Internet, I highly recommend that you speak to *your* doctor about what you can do to improve your chances of getting pregnant. But keep in mind that a perfectly healthy woman in her twenties isn't going to get pregnant every time she has sex, even if she's ovulating right then.

What does that mean practically? Frankly, it means you would be naïve to expect to go through just one IVF cycle and walk away with the baby you want. It's more likely that you will need more than one cycle. A big UK study recently suggested that some couples may need significantly more cycles—as in maybe six—to achieve a pregnancy.[42] Of course, studies like that don't address the amount of money you would need to pay for that many cycles or how long it would take to pull off that many. With all the waiting and testing and scheduling of infertility, you'd be lucky to squeeze four IVF cycles into a year. If you have miscarriages? Maybe two.

None of this makes it feel better when a frozen IVF cycle fails. But maybe take from it that you should reset your expectations around success and ignore your dear relative who wants you to "keep trying" until you have that baby. No matter how well that person means, they have no idea what you're up against. You're the only person who knows how long you can continue fighting the odds. You're the only person who knows when you need to stop.

INFERTILITY LESSON #8

It's natural to want to know how much you'll have to go through to get that baby you want, and it can be frustrating, and even unbelievable, to learn that you could sink thousands and thousands of dollars into infertility treatments and never emerge with a baby.

I think promises are unreliable in the infertility game, but if you want more information about your odds of success, here are the do's and don't's I recommend:

1. Do talk to your doctor about your particular chances of success and what you can do to increase your odds. Your doctor is the person who can give you the most reliable advice.

2. Don't rely on Google to decide for you if you're likely to have IVF success. *Definitely* do not rely on fertility message boards where anyone can post anything without having any real information or background.

Also, don't rely on your friend, whose doctor told her something that you and your friend think probably applies to you. Your friend's doctor hasn't seen you and doesn't know your particular situation. Plus, different doctors explain things in different ways. By all means, compare stories, but don't assume that what your friend's doctor says to her will have anything to do with you.

3. Do switch doctors if you don't feel you can trust yours. Personally, I dislike both over-confident and under-confident doctors. I want a realist when I ask for medical advice, not someone who will give me all doom and gloom and not someone who puffs up the truth to make me feel better, either.

You could be different from me in that respect. That's okay. You have intuition that will tell you who you can and can't trust. If your gut tells you that the first doctor you go to isn't giving you what you need, see if you can switch doctors. There are likely to be other doctors at your clinic or other clinics in the area. Get a second opinion.

4. Don't expect any doctor to be able to predict the future or guarantee success. They can't. They are doing the best they can with the information they have and modern medicine. So exception to recommendation three: if your "gut" wants someone who can promise you a baby in nine months, you may want to check that gut!

5. Do research your fertility clinic. You can look up the statistics on IVF success for your own fertility clinic on the Society for Assisted Reproductive Technology (SART) website here: https://www.sart.org/clinic-pages/find-a-clinic/.

FINAL THOUGHTS ON FROZEN CYCLES

Most importantly, when it comes to IVF, you need to understand that it's hard to keep doing one cycle after another. What's your limit? When do you decide that you can't take more? When do you need a break?

Those are very difficult questions to answer, and anyone who has a list of easy ways for you to decide when to stop is probably misguided. Making a baby is complicated. Only you know what you and your partner can take in terms of money, time, physical energy, emotional capacity, etc.

Every cycle will take a little more out of you. If you decide enough is enough, let yourself off the hook for making that decision. If you decide you can keep going, do it. This is your life. Only you know how much frozen hell you're willing to walk through to keep trying for that baby.

PART III
Life Without Babies

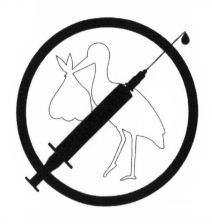

*I can't imagine being that nosy, like,
"When are the kids coming?" because who
knows what somebody's going through, who
knows if somebody's struggling?
~ Chrissy Teigen*

CHAPTER EIGHT
Your Marriage Must Improve

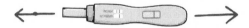

THE BOOTY CALL

It is winter 2018, and we're back at the fertility clinic again in Georgia. We have run through all our eggs and embryos from the first egg retrieval. If we want to keep trying, we probably need to start again with another fresh IVF cycle. We dread having to start fresh.

Mostly, when I'm "between cycles," I am on birth control. This is something that mystifies my family, my friends, and even my primary care physician and ob/gyn. Being on birth control means no hope of getting pregnant whatsoever, right? Almost everyone knows someone who got pregnant naturally after trying IVF. So why am I on birth control?

I'm on birth control because a doctor at the fertility clinic told me I needed to be on birth control. The conversation occurred after my miscarriage in 2015. He told me that no, my periods would not start if I stopped birth control, and it would be better for my uterus to stay on birth control between cycles. I have a love-hate relationship with birth control, but mostly, being off birth control tends to have negative consequences that I can see on my body. So, if the fertility clinic thinks birth control is important to keep my uterus healthy, I'm staying on it.

At the same time, I would now like some chance at pregnancy. So after our last IVF cycle in 2017, I did not go back on birth control. As expected, my periods never started, so being off the pill isn't going to help me get pregnant. Still, when we return to the fertility clinic in February, we ask our current doctor if there is anything we can do between birth control and IVF that would give us some chance. She suggests maybe we should take a step back and try Clomid and timed intercourse again. Those cycles might not work, but they would be inexpensive and low risk. Something easy to give us a shot.

The doctor says I might not need those two weeks of birth control to start the Clomid if I'm already at a baseline level of hormones. So I go to the clinic one morning for bloodwork and a pelvic ultrasound to see where I might be in a cycle, and in the meanwhile, Malcolm flies out of Atlanta for a short business trip. There's an all-firm meeting in Indianapolis that he needs to attend. We assume this will not conflict with our cycle because we assume we have at least a few weeks until I'll be ovulating with Clomid.

We should know better. We should be assuming that the second we don't want my body to do something like ovulate, it will. In the afternoon, I get a call from the nurse. I'm ovulating. Like, right now. The nurse says we need to have sex as soon as possible.

But I am in Atlanta, and Malcolm is in Indianapolis.

If I ovulated regularly, we'd probably just consider this

a missed opportunity, but I hardly ever ovulate. As far as I know, this is the first time I've ovulated without help in years. I call Malcolm, and we agree that we can't just ignore this. So I book an expensive last-minute flight, pack a bag fast, beg my dog walker to please come by early in the morning to make sure our doggie (who is mostly potty pad trained) still has water and is okay. Then I get in my car, drive to the airport, board a plane, and fly to Indianapolis.

It is evening by the time I get there. About seven o'clock. I'm worried that we've already missed our opportunity. An egg doesn't have a long shelf-life. It's only going to be good for twenty-four hours, and sperm need time to reach an egg. From my perspective, we need to get this "timed intercourse" over with ASAP. Hours count, people.

But I'm grouchy because I haven't eaten anything most of the afternoon, and my husband is grouchy because he was supposed to be meeting up with a colleague tonight. He doesn't want to drop everything and "do it."

We go to the hotel bar and order food. Luckily, the bar turns out to be a pretty cool wine bar. It's a little like a Dave & Buster's for winos. You buy "tokens" at the actual bar, the bartender gives you an empty glass, and you then go around the room, redeeming your tokens at various token-operated taps for sample-sized pours of wines. They have all kinds of choices from all over the world.

It is a wine-lover's hotel bar dream, and Malcolm and I both love wine. We have since we honeymooned in Argentina and discovered the magic of a wine tour. We are both stressed tonight, so even though I'm freaking out about timing, I try to enjoy the cheese platter we order and our wine token experience.

Still, minutes are ticking by, and I'm here for sex, not

alcohol. When Malcolm's colleague shows up and Malcolm tells him to sit down with us, I get nervous. We don't have time to spend hours catching up with an old friend. Not right now. We have other business to accomplish.

Malcolm does not seem to share my anxiety. I begin to get angry as he drinks and chats with his colleague like he is oblivious to why I am here. Does he not understand? No, we don't need more tokens. No, we don't need to order a bottle of wine. No, we don't need more food. We need to tell his colleague goodnight and get to the hotel room.

Side note: when I read this to Malcolm recently, I discovered that he did *not* understand. He had no idea our window of opportunity was that slim. But that night, the more anxious I become, the more stubborn Malcolm gets about not ending the evening with his colleague early. It is nearly eleven before we make it to the hotel room.

By then, I am *furious*. This is humiliating, and I didn't drop everything to come to Indianapolis and sit around in a wine bar with some guy Malcolm knew in law school. I am terrified that we have already lost our chance.

Malcolm is also furious. What he wants is for us both to be able to relax and enjoy the sex. I do not see how this is even possible. Timed intercourse is never fun or romantic. We both hate it. I will be tense, which is likely to make it painful for me. He will be tired, and that will make it difficult to accomplish. Plus, we have both had enough wine by now to be high-strung and ill-tempered. The sex we're supposed to have tonight will probably be some of the worst sex we ever have.

A fight ensues. It is a relationship-damaging fight. Infertility has done this to us. We are harder on each other than we used to be. We say cruel things. I raise my voice. I accuse him of not loving me enough. Doesn't he even care about having children? Why can't he ever prioritize his family? Why can't he just cooperate?

He stares coldly at me and says maybe we should get a divorce.

I toss threats like that out far too frequently myself, especially when we're drinking. I seldom mean it. But Malcolm rarely says things like that, and when he does, I think he means it.

I am crushed, hurt, enraged. I feel like I've wasted a whole day here. No, a whole month. No, it's much worse than that. We've wasted tens of thousands of dollars trying to have babies. I've wasted my body with hormones. The toll infertility has taken on my relationships and my career has been one big waste. Hell, maybe our entire marriage has been a waste. If I had known I would go through all that just for my husband to leave me on a terrible night when my stupid ovaries decided to work, I would never have married him.

I start to cry, and he doesn't care. That's how angry we both are. At first. But the truth is, we're both having a shitty day and a shittier night. He eventually apologizes. So do I. No one actually wants a divorce. We don't want what we have right now, but we don't want to leave each other.

Don't think that our "timed intercourse" becomes make-up sex here. Make-up sex is enjoyable. Or at least passionate. What we have to get through is exhausted, emotionally drained, miserable sex. Also, we're both still angry. But we manage it, then we sleep.

If there is one day I would like to erase in my infertility history, that is the day. Not surprisingly, the cycle doesn't work. The pregnancy test is negative. Maybe we were too late with the sex after all. Maybe we were too stressed at that point for my body to decide that, yep, this would be a good time for a fertilized egg to implant. Maybe we were just unlucky again. Doesn't matter. It didn't work. All that effort—and that huge fight, too—only served to hurt our relationship.

I would like to tell you that was rock bottom for us and that we fixed everything the next week. We moved on to IVF feeling hopeful and happy with each other. We never had another fight. That would be a lie. The day after that booty call, we were simply lucky not to be divorced.

But what isn't a lie is that there's something about learning how to face a huge challenge like infertility together that helps a couple grow stronger. You're kind of war buddies after so many years, and there's a loyalty that inspires. It's not luck that's kept us together for the last decade.

FREQUENTLY ASKED QUESTION

My partner and I are going through infertility treatments, and I feel like we never have sex anymore. I'm worried this is going to end us. What can I do?

ANSWER: YOU MUST LOVE BETTER THAN A FAIRYTALE

Before Malcolm and I got married, we met with our minister, a Scottish Presbyterian reverend with an appreciation for scholarship and scotch. He asked us various questions about what we wanted in the ceremony, how we felt about marriage, etc.

We'd just done the church's premarital group counseling

training a few weeks before, and we'd basically failed. We'd learned that we are a "high-conflict couple," and our lack of communication skills was likely to lead us to divorce.

We chose to ignore that premarital advice. After all, we were both *attorneys.* Litigators, even! I had strayed from litigation to become a negotiation trainer and focus on soft skills, but that never helped our relationship much. You try resolving an argument with, "You're not listening! And these are the five tools you must use to make me feel heard." Talk about the opposite of helpful. Malcolm and I were primed to be in a high-conflict relationship.

Still, we did learn two useful things from premarital counseling. First, we learned we should hold hands if we're going to say nasty things to each other. This still amuses us both. We'll say, "the church told us to hold hands!" whenever things get heated in a fight and someone is about to say something awful.

Second, we learned that we're both stubborn as hell. Turns out that Malcolm and I both respond to "you're going to fail at this" with a hearty "screw you." We decided the premarital counselors simply didn't understand us, and we didn't stress over it.

But, when we met with the minister, we realized that we were, perhaps, a little strange as a couple. Had we somehow started our relationship disenchanted with love? We told the minister that we were not one of those couples that were "crazily in love."

"We're not a fairytale," I remember saying. The rest of this I'm paraphrasing, but I continued with something like, "We're not with each other because we can't live without each other. We're with each other because we want the same things out of a life together, and we're committed to doing hard work to make that life happen."

The minister did not seem to think our relationship was likely to end in divorce based on that. Still, there were times early in our marriage when I think we both wondered if we'd screwed something up with love. Other couples seemed so crazy about each other and so proud of that. Had we done this wrong? Was love supposed to be obsessively, crazily needy? Maybe it's not good enough to think the other person has an adorable butt, admirable confidence, a kind heart, and a sexy brain. Maybe you're just supposed to want sex with the other person every hour of every day. Maybe you're supposed to be infatuated to the point that you can't spend a day apart.

We were never like that, and from my perspective, that was by choice. I'd had "infatuations" as a young woman. Those relationships never worked out, and I always left feeling like I'd never been in love with the guy anyway. Maybe I'd been in love with the idea of the guy, but it was usually because he had traits I wanted in myself. I fell for creative, rebellious guys who weren't afraid to be themselves. Took a while for me to realize how needy that was.

By the time I dated Malcolm, I wasn't that needy anymore, and I'd spent a lot of time shedding false skins so that I could be a truer version of myself. Malcolm met me as a creative, rebellious person, and I had no desire to be like him. We were both litigators at big law firms, but I didn't want to be a partner. I wanted something else. I liked Malcolm for his work ethic and his confidence and that butt, but I didn't want to be him. I wanted him to like me, I wanted him to complement me, but I didn't need him to "complete" me.

Today, that sounds like exactly the kind of relationship I would advise a young person to look for, but back when we were dating, it sometimes felt like it must not be sufficient.

Since we could also get in impressive, blowout fights, we both worried that we weren't right for each other.

Malcolm would sometimes say to me, "I'm worried I don't make you happy enough. I'm worried you don't love me enough." I would say, "It's not your job to make me happy. And maybe I don't love you like Cinderella loved Prince Charming, but those fools ended up divorced after they realized there is no such thing as happily ever after. I love you more every day. Isn't that better than fairytale infatuation?"

Yes, I can see why that might sound terribly logical and unromantic, but I always believed I'd be vindicated someday. Malcolm loved me enough to stick it out, and I think maybe I have been vindicated. Our marriage has survived two out-of-state moves, three job transitions for him, multiple entrepreneurial ventures for me, serious depression and anxiety, timed intercourse, multiple miscarriages, and years of not being able to have babies.

We still have fights, but it seems like more time passes between fights now, and the fights we have are shorter and easier to get over. There are lower stakes. We're kinder to each other between fights.

After our most recent move and a second miscarriage, we had this fight where Malcolm said something pouty like, "Maybe we were just *never* right for each other."

I had been saying all kinds of witchy things during that particular dispute, and in response to that, I screamed something like, "What are you talking about!? We're *great* together!"

He started cracking up. I started cracking up. We apologized and agreed that yes, we are great together, because you *must* have something good going for your relationship if you can be a high-conflict, anti-fairytale couple who somehow makes it through what we've made it through. We're *brilliant* together. You will never convince me otherwise. And I still think Malcolm has an adorable butt.

But this is not to say that you need an imperfect relationship to get through infertility hell. It's to say that no matter where your relationship starts, fairytale or not, you will have to get better as a couple once you start going through this. Infertility can destroy your sex life, demolish your expectations about a happy ending, throw anxiety and depression right up in your face even if you've never experienced it before, and mess with all your plans.

It's not good enough to assume love and passion will keep you together through that, unless you think of love as a verb and passion as something you apply to the things you're working for together as a couple.

We're not relationship experts. God knows we still have communication issues. We think we've picked up a few helpful hints, though, especially as they pertain to infertility. So the following is what we recommend to couples going through the infertility slog. Take from this what you think will work for you, and good luck. You're going to need it.

INFERTILITY LESSON #9

1. Rewrite your identity as a couple without kids.

Think about what you and your partner dreamed about having together when you first fell in love. Maybe you wanted to save up for a house, have two kids, work hard during the week, host backyard barbecues with your friends on Friday nights, take your kids to soccer practice on Saturday mornings, then go to church and grandma and grandpa's house on Sunday. Maybe you wanted to build up a nest egg, retire early, and one day watch your kids have kids of their own.

But now you're facing infertility, and you and your partner are both seeing the future you planned washed away. That happily-ever-after is so far in the distance it doesn't even seem possible to get to anymore. It might not be. So who are you now that your dreams are shattered like glass on the floor all around you? Where does it leave you when you were building your whole world around a future you expected to be able to reach?

Answer: it leaves you in the present, learning to love each other in the moment. You can't be about what happens tomorrow anymore. You have to be about what happens today. So you have a choice to make as a couple. You can sit around telling each other how bad you have it, how unfair this is, how jealous you are of your friends and their perfect families, how all your dreams are gone. Or you can say to each other, "Well, since we can't base 'us' on what we'll be tomorrow, what can we be today? What can we do to enjoy each other right now? What can we do to take advantage of our current, childless state?"

Malcolm and I love to take long drives out to small towns and explore local coffee shops, cafes, boutiques, and bookstores. When we can steal time from our work, we love extended road trips, and we do things on those trips that you can't do easily on a "family" vacation.

We rented a car in Italy several years ago and cruised from Milan to Tuscany. We saw opera in Venice and randomly stopped at a five-star Michelin restaurant that happened to have a table for two available for dinner. We popped into a violin maker's shop in Cremona, home of Stradivarius and Guarneri, and Malcolm impressed the shopkeepers playing one of their violins. We drove into downtown Florence, miraculously managed not to hit any pedestrians, and took a cooking class and a wine tour. Then we spent our last few days in Tuscany, sipping wine and eating too much. That's not a trip you take with a baby in tow. Or if you do take it, you probably don't have quite as much fun as we had on those wine tours.

We spent two weeks out west more recently, participating in a car rallye (that's the right spelling!) from Salt Lake City to Santa Fe. We drove the Triumph roadster we eventually replaced our Spitfire with—a 1974 TR-6—leaking oil and without airbags. We kept the top down almost the entire time. We navigated back roads with a group of other vintage car enthusiasts, and we made stops at tiny bed and breakfasts, boutique hotels, small towns, and national parks.

At Zion National Park in Springdale, Utah, we put on our hiking boots and hiked a trail that led us up to a view of the whole park. At Arches National Park in Moab, we made it to the Delicate Arch. Also, our car broke down, and Malcolm spent the afternoon cussing about the car at an auto shop in Moab while I found a local bookstore and an ice cream place. We had to leave our TR-6 behind in Moab and rent another car—one with airbags—for the rest of the trip. Could we have done any part of that trip with two little kids? I don't think they make car seats for 1974 British roadsters.

We acquired a love for Cabernet Sauvignon in Napa Valley, where we've taken great cooking classes and sampled lots of wine that we later shipped home in cases. We spend many evenings trying to replicate great meals we've had in places we've traveled. Malcolm is the chef, and he has mastered everything from Argentinian-style steaks to Florence-style Bolognese sauce. I am the baker, and I've experimented with everything from tiramisu to baklava.

We recently learned how to make beer batter and deep fry pickles together. We love a good "grazing" night with a bottle of red wine, which we can share while we sit outside and talk in front of a fire in our chiminea. We never have to worry about how late we stay up or who needs to be put to bed or who won't like the interesting food we're trying or who is going to start asking "are we there yet?" on a road trip. We are free to be foodies, winos, and car people. That's who we are as a couple.

Does this mean we don't wish we could just spend our vacation money on an overpriced family trip to Disney World? No, of course not. Do we wish we had kids who would keep us from sleeping in on a Saturday morning? Yes. But that's not our world, and for now, we find that we're much happier if we focus on what we can enjoy instead of wasting time wishing we lived in some other world. Surprise benefit? This makes us more interesting people. Lots of couples our age are taking their kids to Disney. Hardly anyone is driving a rallye in an old, tiny car in Utah.

You, too, can have an identity as a couple that doesn't revolve around kids. You just have to be open to the idea and start looking for it.

2. Beware of clinical depression.

If you try to find ways you can be happy and it just seems like happiness is out of your grasp, or if you find yourself doing self-destructive things—drinking too much of that red wine, not being able to fall asleep and sleeping in much too late, getting in petty fights with your partner that turn into blowouts you may not recover from—it is worth considering the possibility that you are living with clinical depression.

Infertility can feel insurmountable, and it's not always

easy to climb out of that pit on your own. If your infertility journey stretches beyond a single IVF cycle, three cycles, five, you could get to a point where you feel pretty hopeless. Even if you aren't the kind of person who would otherwise have been depressed or anxious, you might find yourself slipping to a place you've never been.

If you or your partner are clinically depressed, then gleefully attempting to "find yourself" as a couple without children is likely to feel downright impossible. And you shouldn't assume that if you feel good, your partner does, too. Just because you're a couple doesn't mean you will cope with this the same way. Either or both of you could need some real help.

Malcolm has never experienced quite the depression and anxiety I'm capable of, but I am on a depression drug called Wellbutrin, and I see a therapist regularly. I will discuss this more in upcoming chapters, but you shouldn't ignore it if you or your partner is depressed. If your mind isn't well, it's very difficult to keep your relationship or body well. You need a healthy body and a healthy relationship with your partner to withstand repeated infertility treatments.

So, this isn't a good time to let your pride get in the way. If you or your partner need more than a vacation, a romantic comedy, a Zumba class, or whatever would normally help you cheer up, start looking for a therapist or psychiatrist. You can't be healthy in a partnership if you aren't healthy as an individual.

3. Find intimacy in laughing and crying together.

I once joked to Malcolm that I'd heard some people just have sex and get pregnant. Like it's *easy* for them. He thought that was the funniest thing I'd ever said, and we laughed hard over it. But we understand that's how it works for most people, and before you face infertility, you might also think sex is where intimacy in relationships comes from.

Bad news. Infertility can be a drag on your sex life. Sometimes, this could be because you aren't allowed to have sex at a certain time in a cycle. Sometimes it could be because you *must* have sex at a certain time in your cycle. Possibly it will be because you're doing timed intercourse cycles, and that sex is absolutely awful. Whatever it is, you can bet that infertility will put you in a situation where you only ever want to have sex when you shouldn't have it.

Additionally, a lot of infertility treatments are physically uncomfortable. The bloat and constipation you experience while you're plumping up your ovaries before an egg retrieval is not at all sexy. The irritation you feel because you're taking three estrogen pills a day is also not sexy. Nor is it sexy to have bruises all over your butt from weeks of progesterone shots. Oh, and when those hormones make you hungry and fatigued and you gain weight, it is very hard to feel sexy.

If all of that weren't enough to put a damper on your sex life, there's also grief and depression to kill your libido. Even if you're coping just fine, it's still hard to want sex when it's going to remind you that you're failing at the basic reproductive purpose of sex.

All this means you could be in for some very long dry spells. Maybe one day, I'll write a book about getting your spark back as a middle-aged person with wrinkles and flub. For now, let's just say that if you were only with your partner for the sex, you're in for a nasty shock.

But I bet if you look one level deeper, you'll find that you were with your partner for more than the sex. You weren't in this just to have kids, either. Maybe you haven't thought of it this way in a while, but you didn't commit to your partner just for the good stuff. You committed for the bad stuff, too, like infertility.

There is intimacy in recognizing that you don't have to face this alone, though. You have a built-in support person doing this with you. Someone else is going through the same experiences you're going through, albeit from a different angle. You and your partner are taking those hits together.

So let yourself cry in your partner's arms over your shared grief sometimes. There's intimacy in that. It's a bonding experience to hold that pain together. It's not the bonding experience you hoped you'd have over the baby you wanted to hold together, but it's still your heart and your partner's in the same place at the same time.

Likewise, there is intimacy in learning to laugh together, despite the pain. This is a good time to develop your sense of humor as a couple. You got together initially because you shared at least a *few* things in common, right? Well, sharing an outlook on what makes you belly laugh is something that can get you through hard times.

Don't force yourself to take every moment of pain seriously together. You need times when someone says something about the misery of IVF and it comes out so funny you both laugh until you hurt. You need dirty jokes, inside jokes, snarky jokes, jokes of pure joy. All of that is bonding, too. All of that is you two giving each other permission to have fun even when it feels like you're walking through a sewer together. All of that is intimacy.

I know this sounds trivial, but I believe that for me and Malcolm, finding opportunities to laugh together at home, even on days when we were so sad, helped us learn more generally how to find the light in the dark and the humor in the hard times. That turned out to be a critical tool for constantly going back to a fertility clinic, repeatedly experiencing failure, and not developing trauma around it.

Humor is a healthy defense mechanism when you're spread out on a table with a torture device stuck up you, and your doctor says, "This might hurt." Laughter releases hormones that make you less stressed. It relaxes your body. It helps you take more pain than you otherwise could have taken.[43] It prevents you from clenching everything and making it all that much worse.

I'm not saying you need to learn to "laugh off" a miscarriage. You don't need to be a sad clown. Still, gallows humor can get you through things you didn't think you were strong enough for, and Malcolm and I both see the gallows humor we've acquired as a mark of the armor we've built up. It helps us brace for bad times.

Sometimes we laugh through tears. Sometimes our laughter turns into tears. Sometimes we laugh instead of cry. That's all better than just crying, though. It keeps us tough enough to keep up the fight, and doing it together always draws us closer.

So look, infertility might hurt your sex life, but I encourage you not to let that hurt your relationship with your partner. The emotions you're going to experience as you go through your infertility journey will be so much deeper than any pleasure you experienced with your partner during sex. You will feel joy and pain, and if you allow yourselves to experience that together, you'll pick up intimacy many couples never have. Embrace that, knowing that it is just as intimate to be able to cry and laugh with your partner as it is to have sex, and your relationship will be stronger than ever.

4. Get a dog.

Finally, if you are inclined to pet ownership, we highly

recommend that you get yourself a pet to lavish all your attention on as a couple. Pets, like laughter, are natural stress relievers with a gazillion health benefits.[44] Snuggling a fluffy, furry creature with a wiggly butt, a swishy tail, great big eyes, and kisses to spare can give you joy when nothing else does.

Having a dog also helps make a couple feel that they are part of a family, not just a partnership. When you love a pet together, there's not just me and you. There's me, you, and the dog, and that little trio is the family you have while you're trying to add a baby to the mix.

Malcolm and I got our dog just before we got married. She is our spoiled princess, and we love that dog more than just about anything. There have been many times when we were angry enough at each other that maybe someone would have walked away if it had been just us two humans in our family. Then the dog would stare up at us, like, "But how are we going to snuggle as a family if you don't live together in the same house?" and it would remind us of all the things we want together.

Unfortunately, you will never find a dog as good as ours. It's impossible. Sorry. God only made one of her, and that dog chose us. But we're sure there are dogs out there that are *nearly* as good. (Maybe a cat or two, also, though we are not cat people.) Get a pet of your own, love it like crazy together, and let that love turn you into a family.

FINAL THOUGHTS ABOUT LOVE

There's a reason stories about infertility are featured in the Bible and ancient mythology. Infertility is ugly and scary, and for most of human history, it's been tough on relationships. This is not for the weak.

But if you can adjust your expectations and turn to (and not away from) your partner for support, you may find that your relationship improves. Let that happen. Make it happen. You need your partner right now, and your partner needs you.

P.S. As I finish this chapter, Malcolm has just come into the room to say, "You know what I'm glad we did? Hike up to the Delicate Arch. That was a fun day."

I respond, "It was. Even the part where your jeans ripped in the back while you were at the auto shop."

"Remember how that German woman made fun of me for my boxers being exposed the whole way up to the arch?" Malcolm says. "People come from all over the world to see the Delicate Arch, and we got to do that."

We got to ɗo that. We had that day, which was both the best and worst day of that trip, and what we remember now is that the car broke down, Malcolm tore the seat of his pants, and we hiked to one of the most beautiful things we've ever seen. Together.

I can tell you truthfully that all our best and worst days are like that now, and that's not because we were so amazing as a couple initially. I don't believe Prince Charming and Cinderella would have survived infertility. But we can, because infertility has taught us how to get through the best and the worst together with grace and humor, and we love each other more every day because of it.

We can get through anything together.

(And we *have* had to get through worse, by the way, but *that* is another book.)

CHAPTER NINE
Your Family Must Get Over It

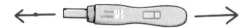

SANTA IS FOR BABIES

It is Christmas of 2016. We are still living in Georgia, and Malcolm's job is keeping him very busy, so we invite our families to spend the holidays with us. They oblige. Both our sets of parents drive from Michigan to see us. My brother and his fiancée fly in from Maryland. My family fills up our guest rooms, while Malcolm's parents get a hotel room. I have an aunt and uncle in the area, and they come to spend Christmas Day with us as well.

It's exciting and a little stressful at first, then it becomes stressful and not-so-much exciting. Mostly this is for reasons that our families do not understand. First, it's the Christmas morning pajamas. For years, my mother has given my brother and I matching PJs on Christmas Eve so that we can open gifts in our matching PJs Christmas morning.

This year, my mom has PJs for me and my husband as well as for my brother and his fiancée. But Malcolm and I aren't into it. I feel like we've outgrown this tradition, and Malcolm thinks the tradition is silly. More importantly, the Christmas PJs remind us that if we had babies, *they* would be in the PJs on Christmas morning and we could be wearing normal person clothes.

For my brother and his fiancée, who are not facing infertility, wearing the Christmas PJs is just a cute throwback to childhood. For me and Malcolm, it is emotionally draining and very sad. We are almost two years past our first miscarriage, and our infertility treatments are still stalled because that's how much that miscarriage affected us. Anything that reminds us that we can't have babies hurts. But my mom loves Christmas, and I feel bad about hurting her feelings by rejecting the PJs. We suck it up and wear them.

We also suck up sitting on the floor of the living room on Christmas morning and pulling little gifts out of the Christmas stockings Malcolm's mom prepared. This is where Malcolm's family does the same thing to us that my family does. Those stockings are not normal stockings. They are huge. Almost two feet tall and nearly a foot wide.

They are also stuffed with the kinds of things you stuff stockings for children with. We get candy and Lego sets and little trinkets. The things we would have put in stockings for our children, if we had children. But we don't. So we have to sit there in our Christmas PJs opening our Christmas stockings like we are five-year-olds, trying to smile like this doesn't hurt.

Then we have to deal with the enormous number of gifts under the tree. Though actually, there are so many gifts that they won't all fit under the tree. Both my mom and Malcolm's mom seem to get a huge amount of pleasure from wrapping tons of gifts and then watching us open gift after gift after gift. It's like they think we still judge whether it was a good Christmas based on the number of gifts we receive. We are thirty-five-years old. We're a little old to think Christmas is all about gifts.

Malcolm and I drink mimosas to deal with this. It is all we can do to get through it. It's okay, though. What I'm looking forward to the most is cooking the holiday meal. I feel like being able to cook a Christmas dinner is sort of a rite of passage. It's something women do when they're grown up and have families and houses. I don't have kids, but today I do at least have the house and a lot of family to cook for. This is something I really want to do.

But cooking dinner quickly becomes stressful, too, because no one seems to understand what this means to me. I keep getting asked what I need help with, as if cooking a meal is too much for me to handle. I don't need help with anything. In fact, not only do I not need help, I do not *want* it. You know what's more stressful than cooking a holiday meal you've been looking forward to cooking? Supervising a bunch of people in your kitchen who think you might need help making gravy.

I tell everyone I would really appreciate if they'd just sit on the other side of the island from where I'm cooking, relax, drink wine, and chat with me while I stir things and put stuff in the oven. My guests cannot handle this. They trample all over my boundaries, and it starts to feel like I'm playing Whack-a-Mole just keeping people out of my way. *Everyone* needs to open the oven and check on something I'm cooking. *Everyone* needs to ask *again* what they can do.

The harder I try to keep the moles out of my way, the more everyone talks about how stressed I am. "Just relax Sandy. We can help!" they say. They do not get that the *foo* is not the problem. The *people* are the problem. I don't need help with the damned mashed potatoes. I'm not a little kid pretending to cook a big dinner. I'm an adult. I can put a frickin' turkey in the oven.

I drink a lot of red wine to get through that. A lot. So does Malcolm, and he is Scottish, so he can drink far more than I can before anyone notices. When people do start to notice that we are both drinking too much, it makes us more stressed, which causes tension between me, Malcolm, and everyone.

At some point during the day (and we do not entirely agree on when this happened, so it might have happened twice), Malcolm pulls me into the dining room and says, "Hey, do you want to just take the car and leave?"

Yes. I really really do. But we can't. We've had too much to drink. We stay, and it's all terribly awkward.

After Christmas 2016, I do explain to my mom and to Malcolm's mom why huge numbers of gifts and Christmas PJs make us feel awful. I have these conversations with them separately. They both cry. It makes me feel like neither of our mothers can handle my efforts to put limits on just how much Christmas grief I can handle. Their grief trumps mine. We do manage to curtail some of the excessive gift-giving and to stop the PJ tradition, but it takes us boycotting at least one Christmas to manage that.

Our families never let us forget Christmas 2016, either. They continue to make little comments about how stressed we were, as if we could not then and never will be able to handle the responsibility of hosting Christmas. If our families come to visit us at Christmas, they try to avoid doing it in large groups, assuming that it was the size of the group that was the problem.

If I get upset because Malcolm's mom decides she needs to cook Christmas dinner in my kitchen, his family thinks it is because I'm being grouchy and difficult. They cannot internalize that maybe taking over a grown woman's kitchen at the holidays could make her feel as though she were being treated like a child, which might remind her that she has no children to cook for.

If my family visits at Christmas, and Malcolm spends most of the day drinking beer and tinkering with his cars alone in the garage, they think it is because he doesn't like them. They cannot comprehend how the explosion of Christmas traditions they bring might remind him that he can't create any traditions with his own kids because he does not have any. They don't get that he needs an escape.

Our extended families get concerned if we don't want to spend time with them at the holidays. They don't think of family events as events that remind infertile couples about how epically they are failing at building their own family. We do our best to find joy in the holidays, but it's not always easy. There's a reason we forget our own birthdays.

If our families asked me what I wanted for Christmas, it would be two completely free things. One, treat us like adults, not little kids, because we desperately need to be allowed to make adult memories of Christmas. Two, give us some grace if we're not on perfect behavior. Christmas might be your favorite time of year, but it is not ours.

No one in our house believes in Santa anymore, and our failure to muster up holiday cheer doesn't mean our personalities are flawed. It means Christmas is hard on childless couples. I have this fantasy where I spend Christmas on a cruise ship, alone, drinking fruity beverages and writing smutty romance novels. Until I have children to celebrate

Christmas with, I cannot think of anything that would make me happier during the holidays.

FREQUENTLY ASKED QUESTION

My family exhibits [X undesirable behavior] about my infertility treatments. I'm so [vulgar f-bomb combo] fed up. I don't think they understand anything about what I'm going through. How do I deal with this?

ANSWER: GREAT FAMILIES STRUGGLE WITH INFERTILITY

So, despite my feelings about the holidays, I would like to say that Malcolm and I come from wonderful families. Our parents would never purposely say something to hurt, discourage, admonish, shame, guilt, or do anything other-wise negative concerning our infertility struggles. All of our parents have said things that have comforted us. My brother always says the right thing. We have awesome extended families, too. The kind you should be jealous of.

We are extremely lucky.

But here's the thing about family and infertility: it really doesn't matter how great your family is. There's always a way for your family to make you feel terrible, and sometimes it happens *because* they're amazing. You can over-love your people. It's a thing.

What I have learned about this from the perspective of the person going through infertility treatments is that most of the time, unless you have an awful family, when one of your family members does or says something that hurts you and the hurt is related to infertility, they have no idea what they have done or why it hurt.

There are a lot of ways your family can hurt you, too. In some ways, your family is in the best position to make your infertility situation seem worse. Let's suppose, for example, that your mom really wants you to have kids. If she asks you if you are still "trying," informs you about some new infertility treatment she heard about, or even just tells you when one of your cousins' babies does something cute, that could all make you feel bad.

Alternatively, let's suppose your mom wants to avoid pressuring you to feel like you must have kids. If she tells you that you are "whole even if you do not have kids," tells you that you shouldn't spend more money on another infertility cycle, or tells you that she thinks it's great that you want to pursue your career instead of continuing to "try," that could all make you feel bad, too.

That's just your mom, though, or possibly your dad or a close sibling. Your family also includes aunts and uncles who might encourage you "not to give up" and might ask you if you're pregnant if you look a little bloated at the family reunion. It includes cousins who don't know how to talk to you when they just had their third baby and you can't have any. It includes your grandparents, who are praying for you to have a baby.

Additionally, no one has to say anything to create a family problem for you. General family expectations could become difficult for you thanks to infertility. Do you have the emotional capacity right now to attend that baby shower? What about your nephew's fourth birthday party? Your little cousin's ballet recital? The family reunion where everyone except you will show up with their children?

How will these events make you feel? Will you have fun? Or will you want to leave halfway through, catch a plane to an island in the Bahamas, and never return to Southeast Detroit again? (That might just be me, but substitute your escape plan there.)

Alas, your family does not suck if they create these problems for you. It's just so ordinary for family to be a source of pain when you're going through infertility. After all, your family was created largely through the act of procreation, and that's what you're failing at. Being with your family inherently reminds you of the thing you can't create like you're supposed to be able to.

Family hurts.

There's just no way around it.

I would like to say I have a lot of tips for how to avoid that hurt. That maybe if you just draw some boundaries and say "no" and tell people what you need, you'll never have a family problem. I don't have that for you, though, and honestly, I don't think that stuff usually works the way you want it to anyway. Not unless you have an absolutely perfect family that is excellent with communication skills and never gets irrationally offended. You can try, but mostly your chances of changing your family are a whole lot lower than your chances of changing how you react to your family and what you allow to upset you.

I doubt anyone has a magic wand that can make this particular aspect of your life better. But here's the advice I do have, some of which might help you deal with your family and the problems they will inevitably create for you.

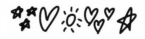

INFERTILITY LESSON #10

1. Expect your family to screw up, and forgive them when they do.

There will always be someone in your family who thinks they are the person who needs to tell you what you should be doing with your body to get pregnant. There will always be a tradition that makes you sad. There will always be a baby you don't want to hold. There will always be a comment or a bad joke that feels like a slap in the face.

Furthermore, your family may not even understand why something they said hurt you. So you could tell yourself that your family members are insensitive jerks who need to learn how to speak appropriately to someone who is going through infertility. But will it really make you feel better to be ticked off at your favorite aunt or uncle because they made a stupid comment? Will it make you feel better if you lecture your grandma about why she needs to stop telling you to keep trying?

It won't. It will make you feel crappy. It's much better if you can remind yourself that the dumb things your family members say and do about your ability to have babies is almost always coming from a place of love. Then let them off the hook and let that stuff slide.

In fact, it might be best if you anticipate that your family will make you feel bad sometimes and tell yourself in advance that you're not going to decide they love you less because of this. Nor are you going to love them less. Family is messy. Infertility is messy. Don't demand perfection here. You aren't going to get it.

2. BUT, don't feel obligated to show up to everything, and call out repeat offenders if necessary.

Since even your family traditions can create problems for you as an infertile person, you may sometimes need to skip a family event. This might be the year you don't do Christmas. This might be the year you don't participate in that baby shower.

Likewise, if it is driving you bonkers that a family member is constantly encouraging you to keep trying, you might have to tell them to stop. You might have to say, "No, we're not sure if we'll ever have kids, we're not sure if we'll try again, and we don't want to talk about it."

Warning: you could bruise some feelings by not showing up to something important. You could make that dear family member feel real bad for saying something incredibly hurtful and offensive to you. So go easy with this. You can always say more later. It's a lot harder to take back something you already said.

At the same time, you may need to be a little selfish about these things right now. If you waste too much energy trying to cope with a draining family event or a family member who always says the wrong thing, you may not have the energy to handle another IVF cycle, another miscarriage, another negative pregnancy test.

So sometimes, you must protect yourself from your family, even when they're the most loving people ever. If they truly love you, they will ultimately understand why you did what you did. They will get over it. They have to.

3. If you are the family member, you need to carry your own sadness.

Family, I know you love the person you are reading this

book for. So if you love them, one of the most important things you can do is distinguish your own feelings from theirs.

Just because you are grieving doesn't mean *they* are. Your infertile family member has probably had to do some serious emotional work to withstand this journey. So, they might be over something you're still struggling with. It's important for you not to make their burden more difficult by adding your bad feelings to what they're already trying to overcome.

This doesn't mean you can't be sad or disappointed when your family member goes through another failed IVF cycle. It also doesn't mean you can't express your sadness or disappointment to and for them. But you need to be careful not to let empathizing turn into you adding your pain to theirs. The difference looks like this:

Your daughter just had a miscarriage. She calls you to tell you, and you cry with her on the phone. The two of you are sharing grief. This is fine.

Two weeks later, your daughter has lunch with you. All you can think about when you look at her is the deep sadness she must be feeling. It is *so* difficult for you not to cry as you think about everything she has lost. This happens the next time you see your daughter also. And the time after that. You notice that your daughter seems frustrated and angry with you when you talk about her infertility. This is because your grief is now a burden for her. This is not fine.

If you get to the point where you're burdening your loved one with your grief for them, it is time for you to find your own therapist or your own self-help book or your own resolution to that grief.

4. If you are the family member, you do not get to decide how far your loved one must go to have children. It's not your call.

You are allowed to want your loved one to have children, but you need to understand that you are not paying the full cost of those infertility treatments. It could get to the point where infertility treatments are costing too much money, too much time, and too much emotional energy for your loved one to take. Infertility could be taking a toll on your loved one's relationships or career. Your loved one might want to move on to adoption.

Since you aren't the one carrying those burdens, it's *never* okay for you to tell your loved one to "keep trying no matter what." It does not matter how much you want grandchildren or how sure you are that your loved one will regret not having kids. When you say, "keep trying," you could be unintentionally telling someone you love to keep holding a heavy boulder over their head. You don't know how close they are to dropping that boulder. You don't know what they're giving up for this.

You need to let your loved one decide when they can keep going and when they can't because if you don't, infertility could ultimately crush them.

And by the way, you *also* don't get to decide what they *can't* carry. When you say, "I think you've had enough," you weaken someone you love, and that's not okay either. It only makes the burden heavier. It doesn't even matter if you think you know what your loved one is going through because you've had some similar life experience. Unless your loved one asks you for your thoughts and advice, you shouldn't be offering unsolicited wisdom about infertility. Your wisdom simply may not be right for your loved ones' life, body, family, relationships, etc.

If you struggle with this, try to remember that we're not talking about you telling your sixteen-year-old not to get a tattoo. This is you telling someone who is probably in their mid-thirties how they should handle a major life issue that they are not in any way taking lightly. If that person needs your help, they'll ask for it.

Not every life lesson can be learned by watching others. Some things we have to navigate on our own. Infertility is generally that kind of thing.

5. If you are the family member, no means no.

If your loved one tells you they cannot attend a reunion, a baby shower, a birthday party, or a holiday dinner, you must accept that. If they can't call their aunt/uncle/grandma/grandpa/cousin/sister/brother who always asks about when they're going to have kids, you must not pressure them to call. If they don't want to have lunch with you next week because they're just feeling too down about babies, you must try not to take it personally.

Infertility has a lot of emotional ups and downs, and again, you aren't the person going through it. There are times when your loved one needs space, and that might mean space from family. It might mean space from you. Do not make their life more difficult by failing to be flexible and understanding. If you love this person, give them space.

FINAL THOUGHTS ON FAMILY

Your family is in the best position to say and do stupid things that make your infertility journey worse than it has to be. They are the ones most likely to think they are "supporting" you when they assume that having a baby is your *absolute, highest priority* in life. They are the ones most likely to be oblivious to your depression, your boundaries, your needs and your wants. Their desire for you to have children may blind them to what you're truly going through. And you probably can't easily fix that.

So don't go to that party if you can't take it. Tell them to stop asking you to "keep trying" if you must. But also, forgive them for all the blunders they make. Their mistakes are probably coming from a place of love. Focus on that. Infertility is hard on everyone. There's no need to make it harder by cutting yourself off entirely from the people who love you.

CHAPTER TEN
Your Friendships Must Change

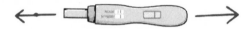

SUNDAY SCHOOL CLASS

It is spring of 2017, it's Sunday morning, and I'm sitting in church where I normally sit. Right side. Two-thirds of the way back. Close to the windows. Next to and behind a group of women who are all at least thirty years older than me. They are wonderful, friendly, kind women who always smile at me and say hello. But I don't have coffee with any of them or call them up to chat. I know very little about their lives.

My husband sits in the choir loft, which is why I'm sitting pseudo-alone. This is a small church, and he has a beautiful voice. The music director found him only a few weeks after we joined the church, and she snagged him for the choir. Because of this, people here started getting to know him pretty fast. His personality is bigger than mine, too. He says hello to everyone, shakes hands vigorously with other men, and seems to fit in naturally to the church's social order.

This, I assume, is why he was asked to be an elder only a

year or so after we joined the church, while people here still barely know me. No one knows *I'm* the one who decides every Sunday that we should even go to church. No one knows *I'm* the one who has considered going to divinity school. How could they? I hardly have any friends here.

But I'm jealous of Malcolm anyway, and I know I probably *would* have friends at church if I could find some way to get to know the women my age. Problem is, they all have kids. And kids change how you are treated socially. The women my age all get called on to mind children after the children's service, volunteer to help at Vacation Bible School, organize the Christmas pageant, and do other child-related things. I'm never asked to do any of that. I don't have kids to talk about or care for. How am I supposed to get to know a bunch of women whose lives revolve around kids?

I have only made one good friend at church so far, and thank God for her. This woman has coffee with me regularly, and we talk about writing, philosophy, politics, theology. We hardly ever talk about kids. She does have children—four, actually—and three are her kindergarten-age triplets. But she's that special mom who seeks out adult conversation that doesn't relate to kids. I don't need any baby experience to chat with her. We're a good match.

I wish there were ten more women like this at church, but there aren't. Women have a tendency to build their lives and their thoughts around their children after they have them. It seems to become difficult for them even to know who they are without their children. There are plenty of things I can talk about if you get me going. We can go mundane, and I can talk about dogs, hairstyles, and homeowner's associations. We can go deep, and I can talk about red wine, books, feminism, and God. (Red wine is definitely a deeper conversation than dogs.) If you're willing to oblige me for an hour, we can even talk about writing. Though most normal humans aren't especially interested in that.

But kids? No. That's not in my wheelhouse.

Malcolm and I did make an attempt to resolve this once. We had a few church couples over for a small barbecue. I don't know exactly what the guys talked about, but the women sat around our table talking about their kids, their kids' schools, their kids' after-school extracurricular activities, and even their labor and delivery stories. I must have seemed like a complete bore. I had nothing to add. Trust me, no one wants you to damper their fun with a story about IVF.

So again, thank God for the one friend I've managed to make who doesn't want to spend our coffee dates talking about kids, but it doesn't really fix things for me at church. My friend happens to sing in the choir, too, and when choir is over, she has to round up her triplets. We're friends on Thursday mornings, when her kids are at school and I'm available to meet up at our favorite local coffee place. Sunday morning, I'm still alone.

I've been attending this church for two years, I love the vibe this place has, I want to make more friends, and yet, I am still an unknown to almost everyone.

Then one day, I'm just done with it all. I don't know what causes me to feel this way, but I'm tired of not being allowed to participate in things other women are participating in just because I don't have kids. I volunteer to be on the Christian Education committee. I know I probably can't run a children's Sunday School class, but maybe I can volunteer at Vacation Bible School or get involved in adult Sunday School.

I do exactly that. I join the committee, and I volunteer to run a one-day adult version of Vacation Bible School. I get really into it. I create an escape room in the church library, and I create an adult version of the children's Bible lesson. I help with decorations and setup. It's fun. I start to get to know a few people.

When VBS is over, I don't want to stop being involved. I volunteer to teach adult Sunday School all year. I have a blast with that class. I talk about controversial subjects. I ask hard questions. We have fantastic conversations, and I start making friends!

I begin having lunch regularly with a woman who is in her eighties. She has children, but they're grown, and she wants to talk about the same things I care about when we get together. She takes me to her writing groups. We talk about politics and commas over pancakes at IHOP. It's amazing.

I find myself going to yin yoga classes with a handful of the women who are my age on Tuesday nights. That's a non-child related thing we have in common. In the spring, I go to a liberal Christian conference with three other women. Malcolm and I start getting invited to game nights with couples who have young children. The kids run around in basements and backyards while the adults play games and chat. Game nights are wonderful for us. They're automatic conversation creators that don't require anyone to discuss diapers, school, or kiddie soccer games.

By spring 2018, we have a whole group of friends. And to my very pleasant surprise, it wasn't that hard after all. I just had to stop expecting anyone to come to me, *Field of Dreams* style.

Of course, we end up having to move from Georgia to North Carolina in summer 2018. And so, the search for local friends begins again. But at least I know what I have to do this time. I start attending writer's groups immediately in North

Carolina, and I organize a feminist book club a couple months after we've settled in. I want to make friends, but these things don't happen on their own. Best to get started early.

FREQUENTLY ASKED QUESTION

My partner and I recently moved to a house in the suburbs. We love our neighborhood, but everyone here our age has kids. How do I make friends with people who have children?

ANSWER: BECOME AN ADULT WHO MAKES FRIENDS

How does *any* adult make friends with any other adult? My theory is that most of them don't. If you take a close look at the adults you know and who they're friends with, I bet you'll learn that, actually, most adult friendships fall into only two categories: (1) people who have known each other for years (i.e. they met in high school or college) and (2) people who met by proximity and have a high number of obvious commonalities (i.e. they live on the same block, are both thirty-two, and both have two young children).

If your friends fall out of these two categories, congratulate yourself. You're a rare bird.

This, unfortunately, is one of the more difficult aspects of infertility. Infertility is incredibly lonely. In part, this is because it's such a personal journey, and your battle wounds aren't clearly visible on the outside. People may know you're going through infertility treatments, but maybe not, and even if they do, you're not shouting about how many doctor's appointments you're going to or what procedures you're having next week. You don't share much of that.

It's also lonely because it forces you to think about a future without the family you envisioned, which probably involved things like children who called you regularly and grandchildren you could brag about. Now that you're not sure you'll be able to have kids, you don't know what will happen to you as you age.

This is especially difficult if your family is already small. I am close to one sibling, and he has no children. My husband is an only child. We don't live near any other family. Because I'm a woman, I'm also likely to survive my husband. If I never have children, that makes growing old a terrifying prospect. Suppose I outlive my husband and my brother. Then suppose I fall and end up in rehab when I'm ninety or develop dementia and need to live in a nursing home. I will move into those places entirely alone. I could die without a single person at my bedside. That's a phenomenally lonely future to be facing.

Of course, children aren't any guarantee that you won't die alone either, but when you have children, you at least have some hope that someone will love you enough to look after you later in life. When you don't, you have to prepare for the opposite. You have to assume that *all* you'll have later in life is the community of friends you built throughout the years.

You need those friendships now, too. You're going through something hard. You need as much support, love, and empathy as you can get from anyone who cares about you. Yet, infertility can strain your existing friendships and make it feel impossible to make new friends. Thanks to infertility, you need friends, and you will also likely have trouble making and keeping friends.

To examine why, let's look at those existing friendships first. There is a gap that splits open when your friends start having kids and you don't. It's natural. You, as someone without children, still have freedom on evenings, weekends, vacations, etc.

But as soon as your friends have kids, they lose a lot of that freedom. They are more tired than they were before. They have to put their kids to bed by nine. They have to pick their kids up from school. They have to hire a babysitter if they want to go out. Brunch becomes a family event. Game night is a family event. Your friends with kids simply can't spend the time with you that they could before.

Additionally, your friends may assume that you don't *want* to be involved in what they see as parental obligations that *no sane person* would want to be involved in. As in, why would you want to hang out at a toddler's soccer game on Saturday morning? Why wouldn't you want to drink mimosas at that amazing cafe downtown instead? Or why would you want to hang out at the park with a bunch of dirt-and-germ-covered-children? Don't you have better, awesomer things to do? Like whatever it was your friends did before kids?

These are reasonable questions. If you want to spend time with your friends, it will likely have to be with them and their kids, and you should probably assume you will have to tell them that explicitly. But sometimes, you might *not* want to spend time watching your friends' kids' t-ball game because sometimes infertility makes attending kid-friendly events emotionally draining.

This all means that you're going to see a change in your existing friendships as your friends move on to "life with children" and you stay at "life without children." It's not that your friends with kids don't care about you anymore. You're simply going in different directions.

What happens with your existing friendships will make it especially important for you to foster new friendships, but that's probably also going to be a challenge. I had a few disadvantages in this area you may not have, but they forced me to directly deal with the challenge.

First, Malcolm and I moved from Chicago to the Atlanta area right before we started going to a fertility clinic, so I had no local friends when my infertility journey began. Then, I moved from the Atlanta area to Raleigh right before we began our second major IVF push, and, again, I had to start that with no local friends. Additionally, my work was primarily contract work that I traveled for during our early infertility years, which meant my schedule was erratic and I didn't work from an office. So, I had no job to use as a springboard to new friends in new places.

Ultimately, these factors forced me to take a pretty close look at the challenge of making new friends, but initially, I made a lot of mistakes in this realm. Probably the biggest was assuming that my peers with children—in my new neighborhood, at my new church, etc.—didn't *want* to be friends with me because *they* never thought to invite me to any social events. It took a while before I learned that women "of a certain age" who do not have kids are often excluded from social circles because they are childless, and yet, this has very little to do with people not wanting to make friends with you.

People who have kids do not intentionally ignore those who do not. However, the social activities of parents do typically revolve around their kids. Parents take their kids to gymnastics, baseball, parks, swimming pools, and museums, not to mention school, church, and grandma's house. The amount of time they have to themselves is limited, and when they get to know new people, it's usually other parents.

It's not a reflection on you as a person if those parents don't invite you to hang out with them. It just isn't going to occur to a woman with a six-year-old that the childless woman two doors down might love hanging out at the aquarium or going to a birthday party for six-year-olds. The two women who spend summer afternoons chatting by the community pool while their kids play aren't going to think to invite a woman who doesn't have kids to join them.

I suspect that most parents even assume it's rude or offensive to invite a childless person to a kid event, especially if they have any reason to think the childless person actually wants kids. They think, "Wouldn't it just make you so sad to attend my baby's first birthday party when you're going through IVF treatments?"

Then let's suppose a brave soul *does* invite you to a play date, a birthday party, a pool party, a trip to a museum, etc., and you reject the invitation. That could easily make the same person think twice about trying again with some other event.

And to further complicate this, you probably don't always want to say "yes" to an invitation like that. If you just had a miscarriage or got another negative pregnancy test result back, you might not want to attend another birthday party or show up anywhere there are children.

That's okay! There are times when you need to control what you're exposed to so that you can stay sane. But a few weeks or months from now, you may really want to be invited to those kiddie events, which are likely to be your only good "in" to making friends with new people who have kids, and it's not going to be easy for the person you rejected the first time to ask again. They're too afraid of hurting you.

So let's sum this all up: adults don't spend a lot of time making new friends with people they don't have a lot in common with. Your existing friends may have less time for you after they have kids and are likely to assume you don't want to hang out with them and their kids. You are, therefore, likely to see a lot of your existing friendships dim. You will need new friends, but anyone in your pool of potential friends who has children is unlikely to proactively attempt to become your friend. None of this has anything to do with whether these people like you. It's all just circumstance.

Are we starting to feel like this is a Sesame Street problem gone all wrong? It is, and if you find someone who seeks out your company even though she has four kids and you have none, you should consider yourself lucky.

But good news. You can fix a lot of this with the folks who have kids and don't think to foster an existing or potential friendship with you. And by the way, I say this as a serious introvert. If I can learn to make friends, you can, even when infertility is affecting you. Here's what has worked for me:

INFERTILITY LESSON #11

1. Keep your existing friends.

Tell your existing friends you would like to be invited to their kiddie events. Tell them you'd love to attend birthday parties, school plays, game nights, picnics, park dates, pool parties, or whatever else they do with their kids that they think you don't want to do.

But also warn your friends that you need to treat this like a meat train at a Brazilian steakhouse. Sometimes, you'll say no to an invitation. That doesn't mean you're offended you were invited. Sometimes, you might ask to stop being invited for a while. Again, this has nothing to do with you being a fragile eggshell friend. You might just need space away from kids when your infertility treatments are getting you down. Explain that it's not personal and you'll tell your friends when the "green light" is back on.

If you have a friend who's going to be hurt or sensitive about your need for social flexibility, they might not be a great friend for you for now. Consider putting that relationship on hold for a while. If you find that you cannot later come back to that friendship, it was probably time to move on anyway. Let it go. It is what it is.

2. Seek out new friends who don't have kids.

Find communities of people whose lives don't revolve around children. They're out there! There are plenty of people who don't want kids at all. I've had my best luck finding those gems in hobby groups, such as my writing groups or book clubs.

You may have to be open-minded. Maybe you thought your next best friend would be a woman your age who lives in your neighborhood, but you meet a woman three times your age who lives with her grown son. Get used to the idea that you can make friends based on common interests, not common age. My husband and I have both made very good friends who fit this category.

3. Be proactive about making friends with people who do have kids.

About those people you'd like to get to know better even though they have kids and you don't: when some brave acquaintance who doesn't know you very well invites you to join a kid-friendly event, don't assume that it was an easy invitation to give. If you can't accept it right now, that's okay.

You don't have to beat yourself up for declining an invitation, and you don't have to give a reason for the "no." But if you think you'd like to accept in the future, you should tell the person who invited you that you appreciated the invitation, that it meant a lot, and that you would like to join in the future.

If another invitation never comes—or if an invitation never came in the first place—it is on you to proactively get involved in social events that you want to be involved in. You may need to volunteer yourself to help with that neighborhood Halloween party that usually revolves around kids. Or you may have to reach out to someone you want to know and invite them over for cocktails.

Remember that adults tend to stick to what they're comfortable with in terms of friendships. They're cliquish. But that's not because they don't want new friends. It's because their friend-making skills are rusty from not being used in a long time. If there's someone you want to get to know better from your neighborhood, yoga class, book club, church, etc., you need to be the person who says, "Hey, do you want to grab coffee with me sometime?" Assume the other person would like to get to know you and assume they won't suggest that latte themselves. You have to be the instigator.

Now, you could be rejected. Honestly, making friends isn't substantially different from dating, and yeah, adults can be total jerks. We aren't kindergartners, and that's too bad because lots of kindergartners are good at making friends. Grown people are far more likely to be insecure, afraid of rejection, socially awkward, and used to being entertained by their phones. We adults have largely lost the art of socializing.

But the upside to all the work you have to do to make friends when you're dealing with infertility is that if you can buck up the nerve to say hello to someone you want to make friends with, you are likely to seem incredibly social and friendly. Not everyone will return your friendliness. Some will, though, and that's all you need. Some. You do not need everyone.

4. If you are reading this as a friend or family member of someone going through infertility …

For anyone reading this book to understand better what a friend or family member facing infertility is going through, if you have kids, please do not be afraid of inviting your childless peers to kid-friendly events. You have no idea what it could mean to that lonely woman who has to watch you and your friends chatting about how hard it is to be parents for you to just tell her she should join you for a glass of wine sometime. The invitation could go like this:

"Hey, Mary and I are getting the kids together next Thursday at the park. I know you don't have kids, but would you want to join us anyway? It's fun. We spend a lot of time trying to ward off injuries, germs, and bruised feelings. Also, we gossip and talk about liberal feminism."

Or that might just be *my* fantasy invitation. You probably have your own. Whatever. Do the invite your way. But don't be afraid to ask.

FINAL THOUGHTS ON FRIENDS

Confession: I was once diagnosed with social phobia. The thought of making new friends was so far beyond me at some point in my life that I hesitated to even include this chapter in this book. What do I know about friendships? I'm not good at this!

Except, I might be a lot better at it than I think these days. Turns out that landing yourself in fertility trouble brings a problem like friendship out in a vivid, bold way. You either have to accept the loneliness, or you have to figure out how to change it. Sink or swim, so to speak. I attempted to make those friends, and I guess I've done it enough times now that it's not as terrifying to me today as it was a couple decades ago.

If you're like me, you might realize you have a little advantage in this realm, too. If you were ever too shy to speak loudly enough to be heard or to make eye contact with people you want to be friends with, that probably means you spent a lot of years just observing how other people behave. I don't know if extroverts do this. But observant introverts eventually notice that most people aren't good at being social. Most people are quite awkward.

So maybe this chapter doesn't apply to you at all. Maybe you're a people-person. Maybe you think it's pathetic to imagine any person—childless or not—feeling lonely and struggling to make friends. It's certainly not something you're worrying about. If that's the case, great. Good for you. Move on to another chapter. But if you're feeling lonely, know that the hard work you have to do now to keep existing friendships and develop new friendships is actually good for you. You'll emerge from this as an adult who can make friends, and that will help you later. Learn how to include yourself now, and you won't be playing bingo alone when you're ninety-five. It's that simple!

CHAPTER ELEVEN
Your Career Must Evolve

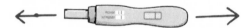

WHAT GAVE FIRST

It is 2008, and I am an associate attorney at my second law firm. I was nearly fired from my first law firm, and I'm not doing much better at the second. Law turns out to be a terrible field for me, and I am considering everything from going back to school to get a PhD (ha!) to trying to find work with a non-profit organization (those jobs are harder to get than you think) to applying to teach English in China.

That last option is where I think my best chance at happiness might lie. I took four years of Mandarin Chinese in college. Only about five years have passed since then, and I still have a few Chinese language skills.

More importantly, I have no idea what I really want out of a career. I went straight through from college to Harvard Law School without any clear concept about what it would mean to be an attorney. I'd have quit law school if I hadn't been going to Harvard. The teaching English in China idea has been rolling around in my head since then. After my first year in law school, I seriously considered taking a year off to do it. I even had a meeting with a school counselor to talk about the possibility.

The counselor thought it was a great idea. At the time, my boyfriend did not, nor did my parents, and I was too afraid to swerve from what I thought was a more "stable" path.

That was a mistake. Maybe the biggest I've ever made in my life. Which, I suppose, isn't that bad. I never did drugs or committed petty crimes. I have no tattoos, no skeletons in the closet. I just went to law school, graduated, and discovered that I hated the practice of law. But it was still a mistake not to take a step back when I should have. Now I am in a job I'm bad at, I'm burdened by a lot of law school debt, and I need out. I am going to drown here otherwise.

My career is a mess.

And right then, I meet this guy. One of my work colleagues introduces us, and I'm not especially into him at first. He seems kind of fancy for me. He has a hyphenated first name. I feel awkward with him. Still, my colleague believes we could be a good match, so I agree to meet John-Malcolm Cox for a first date at my favorite pizza place in downtown Chicago.

Malcolm is also an associate attorney at a law firm, but while I show up for dinner in jeans and wanting to talk about anything but law, he shows up in a suit and tie and tells me it's important to "dress for what you want to be." He wants to be is a partner at his firm. I would rather, well, not die, but at least move to a foreign country and never set foot in a law firm again.

We do seem to have a lot of other things in common— we're Midwesterners, Presbyterians, car people, music lovers—but none of this counts compared to the deep divide between the two of us related to our career goals. Also, there's no way I'm going out again with a guy who aspires to be a partner at a law firm. I mean, seriously? Why would I invite that hell into my life?

We don't see each other again until February of 2009, when I need a date to my church charity ball and Malcolm Cox is the only single guy I know who might agree to be that date. Malcolm does go to the same church I go to, after all. I never see him there. It's a huge church on Michigan Avenue. I really want to go to that fundraising event, though, and I don't want to go alone. Malcolm says he'll come with me, and to my great surprise, we have a good time together.

We start dating. I am honest with Malcolm about where I am in life. I tell him I hate my job. I tell him I am getting out of the law firm world come hell or high water. I tell him I'm not interested in dating anyone who isn't okay with me wanting to travel and live abroad. I tell him I'm thinking of moving to China to teach English.

Malcolm maintains that what he wants is to make partner, but for whatever reason, I think it makes him happy that I'm a law firm rebel. I warn him that it is extremely important to me that I find a partner who will support my dreams. He tells me his law firm has an office in China. We go out on more dates. We have a lot of fun together. I think this is a guy I could spend my entire life with.

We get serious, and a few months before we get engaged, I tell Malcolm I've started applying for those teach-English-in-China jobs. I'm also looking into three or four other programs that would let me work abroad.

My plan makes a ton of sense for me as an individual. I'm saddled with hundreds of thousands of dollars of law school debt, but my Harvard J.D. comes with a great debt forgiveness program. If I'm doing something like working for a non-profit organization teaching English in China, Harvard will pay my debt while I work. I can live off my teaching stipend during that time, do something good for the world, and maybe figure out what I'm truly passionate about, all while an impressive foundation pays my debt.

Hopefully, I can come back and get a master's degree or PhD—which would also keep me covered under that debt forgiveness program—and then I could work in academia later. I think I might like teaching at a university in a subject I care a lot about. I just need to figure out what that subject might be.

There's a flaw in the plan, though. Malcolm told me he could work from his office in China, right? I'm assuming we can take this adventure together, and I expect him to be receptive to what I'm saying since I've been talking about this the whole time we've been dating. But for Malcolm, my job applications are a reality check.

"I can't just work from China," he tells me.

"You told me you had an office there," I say. "Why not?"

"My career is here in Chicago," he says. "I can't move."

This is our first true fight—or maybe you could even call it a power struggle—but many years down the road, I'll see it as the first time I choose my family over my career. Malcolm holds a hard line. I can give up a career dream I've been fostering for years and stay in Chicago with him, or we can break up and I can go live and work wherever I want.

I choose him.

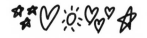

FREQUENTLY ASKED QUESTION

I'm trying to schedule an IVF cycle, but my job needs me more than ever. I'm working long hours and traveling. I have meetings from early in the morning to late at night. My career is important to me, and it is part of why I waited so long to have kids. Once I start the IVF cycle, how will the fertility clinic accommodate my work?

ANSWER: TRICK QUESTION!

Your fertility clinic will have a schedule in the sense that you might have to wait to schedule a consult until a doctor is available or they might only start so many IVF cycles in any given week or month.

However, your cycle's start date is pretty much the only thing you will get any flexibility with, and even that might depend on something like when your period starts. Your fertility clinic might also be able to give you a tentative date for an IVF transfer or egg retrieval. But once that cycle starts, everyone involved is at the mercy of your body. You, your partner, your doctors, your fertility clinic. You will all be waiting on your body and your hormone levels, your ovaries and your uterine lining.

And if you are anything like me, the minute you need your body to cooperate with your work schedule, it will disobey.

In my experience, there is very little flexibility when it comes to infertility treatments. No, you can't reschedule your IVF transfer to the next day if you have a work emergency that prevents you from getting to the transfer the day it was scheduled. No, you can't change when your ovaries are ready for egg retrieval. No, you can't tell your body when exactly to start your period. No, you can't pause your cycle and postpone your baseline appointment to next week. No, you can't even plan the "easier" infertility treatments, like timed intercourse or IUI, with any precision.

You simply can't tell your body exactly when it should ovulate, when your uterine lining should be ready, or when your hormone levels should measure perfect for a potential pregnancy. You have to be available and flexible for a couple weeks instead. So no, you don't get to have a work emergency that takes you out-of-state for two weeks during the middle of a fresh IVF cycle. That could ruin that whole $15,000 show.

Really, the only thing that a fertility clinic can do to help a working woman is to guess how long a cycle might last from start-to-finish and try to avoid scheduling any cycle when the woman is likely not to be available. The two clinics I've been at also try to help by offering early-morning monitoring and baseline appointments so that you can come in to get those done before 9am.

The rest of it is out of their hands and out of yours.

Infertility is hard on a working woman.

TRAVEL RESTRICTIONS

It is somewhere between 2010 and 2017. I'm not really sure when. This is a career story, and those work years run together for me.

During that time, I take on contract work for a negotiation training company. It's a great gig for me career-wise.

I love being a negotiation trainer, and I'm good at it. I work with companies across all kinds of industries and people at every level within those companies. I have lots of autonomy, and I facilitate training all over the world. I've trained negotiators across the U.S. and Canada, plus I've done training in India, China, the U.K., Europe, and Australia.

When I'm not traveling for a training, I work from home, and this makes my work a good compromise for Malcolm and me. I don't have to work in a law firm anymore, but I do get to travel and I get a broad look at a wide variety of businesses, industries, and occupations. I'm never bored.

The downside is that my gigs don't pay nearly as well as Malcolm's job, and there is no debt forgiveness available with this kind of work. I am still contributing substantially to our household income, though, and I at least manage to cover my loan payments.

Malcolm works much longer hours, but this is what he bargained for, too, and the freedom I have at home allows me to take over most of our household business. I pay the bills, walk the dog, do the laundry. Also, when Malcolm wants to pursue career opportunities, my work doesn't get in his way. When he gets a great job offer at a law firm in Atlanta, I can easily pack up and move with him because I can do my work from anywhere with an international airport.

Yet, I have the sense that time is flying by as I rack up frequent flier miles, and while there are slow months for me, there are also months when I'm so busy that I am barely sleeping and perpetually jet-lagged.

Thankfully, the company I work for is small and family-oriented. When I start infertility treatments, I let them know, and they are as supportive as they can be. There are conflicts anyway. The company schedules training jobs anywhere from six weeks to a year out, so if I agree in February to do a training in California in May, I basically put myself in a situation where I can't start an IVF cycle in April or May. This creates huge gaps in time from one infertility cycle to the next, and I don't know how to fix the problem. How am I supposed to do an IVF cycle in Atlanta when I'm conducting negotiation training in London?

By the end of 2016, I realize this is no longer working for me. I'm tired and stressed. I don't look forward to training anymore. I'm thirty-five years old, and I'm feeling a fertility time-crunch. I need local work. I try starting a solo law practice, but I still strongly dislike the practice of law. That's my first entrepreneurial venture, and it's a bust.

Next, I try starting a consulting company of my own with a colleague, hoping that I can build up a local clientele in Atlanta, but it turns out that it's difficult to find local clients who will pay well for training sessions. Inevitably, any time I attempt to be flexible for the sake of a great opportunity with a client, I end up in trouble. One fall, I'm so busy with a Vancouver-based client that I barely sleep for months.

None of this is conducive to infertility, and time is ticking by. I can't keep this up. If I want to get pregnant, I need to step back from my work and focus on IVF.

Then Malcolm gets that job offer to go in-house as an attorney in Raleigh, and the opportunity is too good to refuse. We move to Raleigh, and if I ever had a chance with the consulting company I'd started, this sets me back several steps. "Local" is North Carolina now, not Georgia. If I want to keep pursuing that, I have to start all over building a clientele. I have no idea how couples ever function when both people are entirely focused on their career, especially during a move. When both of your careers are keeping you busy, who's at home with the movers, signing forms, packing things up and unpacking them, minding the dog, hiring painters, waiting for the cable guy to show up, and on and on as you relocate your life from one state to another?

I find this whole question puzzling. If you both have big careers, how do you decide who leaves their job when one of you gets an amazing offer in a new state? I can't imagine saying to Malcolm, "I know you want to take a job in another state, but my work is here. You can stay with me, or you can move." What would he have done? Is it possible that most couples *can't* pull two big careers off at once? Is that why most people don't move as much as Malcolm and I have?

In any case, mine is the career that has to flex in my marriage, so once we get to Raleigh, I have only two reasonable directions. I can try to bring that fledgling consulting business to North Carolina and spend all my energy attempting to build a new local clientele in a city I barely know. Alternatively, I can give up consulting and try to find a full-time job using the skill set I've acquired from training and lawyering.

If we didn't need to get back to infertility treatments, the second choice would probably sound like the right answer. But if I take on a full-time job, my husband and I will have to hire out much of the work I do for our house, and, more importantly, venturing into a completely new career space will mean an entirely unpredictable work schedule.

If you think telling your boss you're pregnant is hard, try taking a new job and then telling your boss that you're doing IVF treatments. Talk about a difficult conversation. If I get a full-time job, we probably won't be able to start IVF treatments again for at least a year. I'm almost thirty-eight now. We do not have a year to put this off.

The one thing I have left that could serve as a source of income is writing. Over the last several years, I've spent my free time learning how to write fiction books. I finally have a finished manuscript that I'm kind of proud of. I'm shopping it around but also seriously eying the self-publishing world.

And remember how I started this story not sure what I truly cared about? Well, writing is something I truly care about. I find that I could write for hours and always want to go back to it again. If I got stuck on a desert island with no hope of ever being rescued, I'd probably write myself stories in the sand, even knowing that the tide would wash them away before anyone could ever read them. Writing could be my passion. It could be my vocation.

My husband and I talk this over at length. The fact that we don't have kids is starting to hit Malcolm hard, and he feels it would be valuable for me to be at home more often.

So, I choose a third path and decide to start writing and publishing full-time as an indie author. I start a small publishing company, and I estimate that it will take three-to-five years of hard work on my writing before I'm making any real money at it. I'll be in the red until then. But in the meanwhile, I can do all my work from home, I can choose my own schedule, and when I need to prioritize my family for the sake of an egg retrieval, I can do that.

That's how I become a writer.

INFERTILITY LESSON #12

You will need flexibility and patience from your job if you want to pursue infertility treatments. This will be difficult to acquire, especially if you want to keep the fact that you're going through infertility treatments quiet. It is incredibly unfair, but infertility could hurt your career.

I hope it doesn't hurt yours, but at some point, if you want to "keep trying," you might be faced with a choice between putting your energy into your career and putting your energy into infertility treatments. You may have to "lean out" if you want babies, and you might have to do it at exactly the time when you need to prioritize your career if you want to build it.

Nothing will get you out of this, either. Not unless you have the resources to outsource everything to a surrogate. Otherwise, the advice other career women get about "just hiring a nanny to be part of the team" or persuading your spouse to take on the burden of housework and childcare won't solve your problems.

This is the kind of gender imbalance that no one bothers to talk about because it is not fixable. Your husband will not need to spend the same hours in the fertility clinic that you will. He will not have the same restrictions you do. If he has to travel or he's busy at work, that won't ruin your cycle. You can go in for those monitoring appointments alone. You can learn to give yourself those shots. But you can't trade places here. Your husband can't do those pelvic ultrasounds for you. That's on you. You're the one whose career has to flex. His will probably be fine.

While you are sacrificing your career for the mere possibility of a family, people will judge you for it. It won't make sense to anyone else why you couldn't focus on your career when you don't even have children. You, like me, could end up in a no-woman's land between being a "stay at home mom" and a "career woman." I often face people who think I'm underemployed because I don't have a full-time job or a stable income of any kind right now. I am entirely reliant on my husband's income. No one knows what I've given up. No one knows I work more hours as a self-publisher than I ever worked in any job. No one knows why I've made the choices I've made.

So when you are deciding if you want to keep pushing forward with more infertility treatment cycles or want to start one to begin with, keep in mind that this will be tough on you if you have a demanding job. Also, be suspicious of anyone who promises that you can have exactly the career you want and the family you want when you're struggling to create that family. Maybe you can, but more likely you can't.

About half a year ago, I had a great discussion about this issue in my feminist book club. A woman several years my senior listened to me complain that it's hard to explain why I am "self-employed" when I have a Harvard J.D. Then she said, "You don't need to explain. If someone asks you why you're not working, the answer is 'this is what my family and I chose, and it's none of your business.'"

I really think she had that spot-on. So, know that there could be difficult choices ahead. Consider the ways your career could bend around your family goals, and be prepared for people to judge your choices. Then, at the end of the day, understand that the big question is: what do *you* want? This is your life. You probably can't have everything, but the choices are yours to make.

FINAL THOUGHTS ON CAREER

You might be thinking here that I have a lot of regrets around infertility and my career. Or maybe you think that I have a lot of regrets around infertility and my family generally.

It's not super-typical for women to say they regret having children, but women do sometimes end up feeling that their decision to have children somewhat hampered their ability to follow all their career dreams. Parents love to say that "having children changes everything," and they say this as both a complaint and a sort of badge of honor.

You know what? Not being able to have children also changes everything, and no, those childless years aren't necessarily a dream for someone struggling with infertility. I had to give up a lot just to stay with my husband in the first place. Then I had to give up more to make two major cross-country moves with him and continue to pursue infertility treatments. I don't have children, and yet, I've closed the door on whole career paths.

Do I regret it?

Not anymore.

I have had times over the last decade when I've lamented things I gave up. But looking back, I always feel like I made the right choices.

Why did I choose to stay with my husband instead of hop on a plane to Beijing? Because I valued the possibility of a family with him more than I valued exploring my potential in a foreign country. I don't think that choice was bad.

Why did I leave my consulting job and opt to try my luck with my own company? Because I couldn't keep up with the travel and still do IVF treatments. Again, I wanted the possibility of a family. I don't think that choice was bad either.

Now, those choices weren't easy. I think sometimes life is molding you in ways you don't realize, though, even when you're going through hard times and making tough choices.

I didn't get to teach English in China, but I did get to use my law degree for many years with the kind of work that let me travel the world, meeting interesting people and learning interesting things. It was exciting and glamorous, and I still enjoy teaching negotiation periodically, especially when I can do it in a virtual context.

When I didn't feel I could travel anymore and do infertility treatments, I used what I'd learned to become an entrepreneur. Entrepreneurship is, of course, an exercise in failing until you succeed. The law practice was a bust. The consulting firm was better but didn't get me exactly where I wanted to be. But the publishing company has real potential, and by now, I've written and published eleven books, including this one. It could take a while before publishing is profitable for me. Still, this venture gives me exactly the flexibility I need, and it's something I love. And I got to this because of infertility.

I didn't realize it while it was happening, but my career evolved around my priorities, and as I went, I was picking up pieces of who I would ultimately become. Everything I did from 2008 to now led me to this life, and I'm quite happy doing what I'm doing career-wise these days.

It's hard to know how infertility will affect your career, and it's hard to sacrifice pieces of your career to infertility treatments. It's hard to make those sacrifices without knowing if you will ever end up with the family you want. You might not have those babies. Then how will you feel about the toll infertility took on your career?

But that's how life works, doesn't it? We make choices based on our priorities at the time, and the choices we make don't always look as good in the rear-view mirror as they did when me made them. Sometimes they look much worse.

Sometimes, they look much better.

Either way, you already made those choices and you can't change them now. So I say, let go of your regrets and focus on the positives of your life choices. Where are you now? What about your life makes you happy? What are you proud of? What did you do that made you who you are today? What are you going to do today to give yourself the tomorrow you want?

Do the best you can, because that's all you can do, and trust that life is taking you where you're supposed to go. Let your career and yourself evolve. You may be surprised one day to learn that all the difficult choices and all the struggles have taken you somewhere you always wanted to be, even though you didn't know it until you arrived. You're going to have to give up some things. You can't control much of anything when you're dealing with infertility. But there's beauty in evolution. Look for that beauty, and let go of your regrets. That's all you can ask of yourself.

PART IV
Managing Grief & Loss

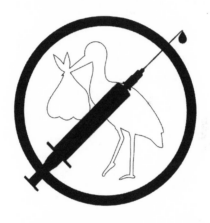

There is no greater agony than bearing an
untold story inside you.
~ Maya Angelou

CHAPTER TWELVE
A Thousand Little Disappointments

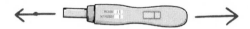

YET ANOTHER NEGATIVE

It is summer of 2017. We've just gone through another IVF cycle, and today is the day of the pregnancy test. It's a Sunday, so we drove to the fertility clinic this morning before church for the test. This made us late to the service, but we need a distraction, so it's better for us to be in church than anywhere else.

Malcolm would normally sit up in the choir loft, but this time, we sit together in the very back row of the sanctuary, just in case the clinic happens to call with our results before the church service ends. It really is a "just in case." Usually the call from the clinic doesn't come until one or two in the afternoon. Today, the clinic is faster than normal, though. We get the call before church is over, and we have to scoot out of our row fast and scurry out of the sanctuary.

I am too nervous to take the call myself. Malcolm takes it. I feel numb while he listens to the news. I can tell it isn't positive. There would be some enthusiasm on his face if it were positive. The test is negative. Another failed cycle.

This is our third IVF cycle and our sixth fertility cycle generally, and I've met women who've done a lot more IVF than we have, but this still stings.

We leave church early. Later in the afternoon, our minister and her husband call us to check in. They tell us they're so sorry to hear about this news. They say things like, "I can't imagine how this must feel. It must be one of your worst days."

We love this couple, and it is extremely sweet that they called. Hopefully, they can't tell from the tone of our voices how we really feel about this. The truth is, even in terms of infertility, this isn't one of our worst days. This is just a negative pregnancy test. Another little disappointment sitting there alongside thousands of others.

FREQUENTLY ASKED QUESTION

I just got the call from the fertility clinic. It's another negative pregnancy test. How many of these can I take?

ANSWER: YOU CAN TAKE MORE THAN YOU KNOW

I don't cry easily anymore. Or maybe that's only half-true. There's this kid's movie, *Rise of the Guardians*, and the scene at the end where the little kid tells the villain, "I do believe in you, I'm just not afraid of you!" can send me into a straight-up sob fest. I'm a sucker for good animation.

But when it comes to physical pain? Emotional pain? No.

Those things don't have the power to make me cry as easily as they used to. My infertility journey has come with thousands of little disappointments. There's always another delay. There's always another negative pregnancy test. There's always another reminder of something I've lost and can never get back. There's an endless buffet of infertility pain to choose from. If I cried over everything that hurt, I'd spend all my time crying.

You can only get cut in the same place so many times before the skin stops healing and you learn to live with an open wound. Or, as I often prefer to think of it, there's only so many times you can get cut in the same place before that skin starts to thicken up. When you go through infertility, there's always another cut.

What's challenging about this, however, is that no one really understands the complexity of infertility grief. Most people prefer to simplify it to make it easy on themselves. They assume that when it comes to infertility, "pain" means "physical pain associated with injections and IVF" and "loss" means "miscarriage" or "lost dreams of the children you hoped to have." So they also assume that once you have a baby, you will have nothing left to grieve. Having a child will meet your ultimate goal and make up for the pain infertility caused and the children you lost before.

Wrong.

First, there's more pain and loss than you expect, and not all of it can be erased by finally having a baby, no matter the means. Having a baby does not make it okay that you lost other babies to miscarriage or stillbirth. It doesn't make you forget about the embryos that didn't implant or the eggs that didn't fertilize.

It irritates the hell out of me when someone responds

to learning about my infertility with, "Why don't you just adopt?" Talk about a clueless thing to say. Adoption isn't easy. You can't just go to the store and pick up a child someone returned. Adoption is expensive, time-consuming, emotionally challenging, and not at all guaranteed.

Furthermore, adoption might get you to "the finish line," so to speak. But there are things to grieve even if you are blessed with an adopted child. Yes, I'm sure if I adopt a child, I'll love that child like crazy. But I'll still have lost the ability to know what a baby my spouse and I created together would have been like. I won't get to see Malcolm's pretty hazel eyes in my daughter's face. I won't get to see my smile when my son laughs.

Whether you later adopt or birth a child, you also lose less tangible things that you can never get back. Time is what I grieve the most. Even if I bring home a baby tomorrow, I've lost so much time with that child! Eight and a half years at least. That's nearly a decade I would have had with that child if I'd had him in my late twenties instead of my late thirties. That's nearly a decade he'd have had with me, with his father, with his grandparents.

I think there are advantages to being an older parent, and if I am blessed with children, I hope I can still manage to be a bright, shiny, energetic parent to those children. Realistically, though, I'll also be a little stiffer, fatter, grayer, and sleepier than I would have been if I'd become a mother a decade ago. Will my child resent that? How will he feel if he wants children and can't have them until he's forty? I'll be eighty by then. Will I still manage to be a spry grandma? Do I have any hope of seeing my great grandchildren at all? Probably not unless medical research steps up our longevity game long enough for me to live well past a hundred.

And there are personal losses, too, even if you eventually have children. I believe that infertility can be a transformative experience that changes us for the better, but that transformation occurs while you're shedding things you once valued deeply. You may lose friends, you may lose career opportunities, you may lose connections you had to family, you may lose your marriage if it's not strong enough.

Those casualties are real, they are not in your head, and finally having children doesn't give much of that back. You have a thousand little things to grieve for as you go through this process, and you're not unreasonable if you resent the people who feel they can cheer you up by telling you there's "still time" and "you won't feel like this once you have kids!" Those people don't get it. They can't. They're only thinking of this from one angle: your goal is to have a baby, and once you have one, you'll have nothing to be sad about anymore.

By the way, I don't think this is an issue you should even bother trying to educate people on the outside about. You basically have to cope with this on your own because frankly, the continual grief you have to deal with during your infertility journey and after isn't grief most people can cope with. The people who love you will be able to handle it if you cry over a miscarriage once or twice while you're with them. We humans like to empathize a few times and then move on, feeling like we've helped our grieving friend carry the burden of the grief and then let it go. But no one wants to know they have a friend who is constantly suffering. We don't want to think that could happen to us.

And what if you never have kids at all? If that happens, you will survive. You'll have to survive with a different set of skills, but you will be okay. However, you'll often have to keep your grief to yourself. Because to the outside world, the thought of someone wanting children and never having them is unthinkable. In fact, it is *so* intolerable that it makes for a great fictional drama. For a while, it seemed to me that every new popular work of literature I picked up was about a woman who had one unplanned pregnancy (but ultimately went on to find joy in life) or a woman who had three miscarriages (and ultimately went insane and stole someone else's baby).

Writers *love* to center their plots on reproductive disasters, and the "woman can't have babies, goes insane" trope is a favorite. Readers love to immerse themselves in the tragic fate of the childless woman, whose fictional mountain of despair is so great that it transforms her not into a wizened, eccentric, well-traveled, wealthy woman, but into a batshit crazy hermit who spends her time watching kids like the witch from Hansel and Gretel.

I'm not sure the true story of infertility is even believable to most people. I once wrote a short story about an infertile couple and submitted it to a contest. One judge loved it. The other two said it was "unrealistic." They didn't think the woman seemed like she really wanted a baby. I guess showing up at a fertility clinic over and over isn't enough commitment and the woman certainly shouldn't have gone on with her life without going insane.

(Screw you, contest judges. You clearly do not know what you are talking about. Also, note to any literary writer considering an infertility plot: the deep grief that results from not being able to have babies does *not* usually turn a woman into a psychotic killer. Please stop perpetuating that myth. It is offensive.)

In any case, my point here is that people on the outside get very black and white about infertility. They assume either you can fix all your pain with a baby, or, if you can't have a baby, they assume your pain is irreparable and you are doomed to a life of misery.

What bullshit. As if there's no gray area where you never have children, and yes, you live with that pain, but no, you do not let it define you. As if there's no way you could eventually have children, love them, be overjoyed by them, and still feel sad sometimes about things you lost because of your infertility journey.

I sometimes wonder how it's possible that so many people can't understand that gray area. My working theory is that everyone hits this pain in some way or another at some point in their life, but until you do, you don't understand that grief isn't black and white. Infertility comes to you at a relatively young age. Maybe that forces those of us who go through it to come to grips with the fact that life is complicated, and you can feel both hurt and hope at the same time. Though I know plenty of people going through infertility who haven't yet figured out that if you want to make the best out of infertility you have to both respect the multiple levels of grief this will put you through and also learn how to let in happiness and joy while you're in the thick of it.

If you're struggling to come to that place, here are things I've found helpful:

INFERTILITY LESSON #13

1. Acknowledge that you're hurting when you experience another loss because of your infertility.
This holds true for big losses and little losses, losses that are contained in time and losses that seem to grow over time.

That negative pregnancy test is a loss. That trip you took with your parents that didn't involve grandchildren they could spoil is a loss.

It is fair and okay for you to feel that pain. Important even. If you don't acknowledge your grief, sit with it, and deal with it, how do you make space for the growth that can come from this kind of personal war? Feeling deep pain is what lets you know what deep joy feels like. Just watch out for the possibility that you're dwelling in your grief too much and not letting in any of the good feelings. You don't want to get stuck with only the bad.

2. Speaking of which ... it is okay to feel loss and hope all at once.

Infertility grief is especially trying because you often have to move right back into a new cycle immediately after a loss. You get a negative pregnancy test, your period starts four days later, and you're calling the fertility clinic that day to get started on your next frozen IVF cycle.

It can seem like you only get a few *moments* to hurt before you have to jump back into something that you're supposed to feel hopeful about. You're swinging like a pendulum between good and bad feelings, and unless you want to delay your next infertility cycle, you don't have time to stop that swing.

So make space for both the good and the bad. Hope and hurt can exist at the same time. Just because you want to be hopeful that this cycle will work, doesn't mean that you can't simultaneously be hurt that the last cycle didn't.

Don't let anyone who thinks you should only feel one way or the other make you question your own gut if you need to feel more than one thing at once, either. You don't need to rush this. Infertility emotions are complex, and there's nothing wrong or crazy about you if you have moments during this journey when you're both intensely sad and intensely happy. It does not mean you are destined to be insane. It means you are human. Humans are complex. Humans are also amazing. We were made capable of having and handling complex, conflicting emotions. Take some comfort knowing that there's no reason you need to force yourself to choose.

3. There is no "right" way to deal with your grief.

Sometimes I cry. Sometimes I can't cry. Sometimes, I'm cool as can be, and sometimes, I want to scream and break something expensive and made of glass.

I'm the kind of person who needs to be allowed not just to feel and acknowledge the full spectrum of emotions but to live out those emotions from time-to-time. When I feel sad and hopeless, it doesn't help me to pretend like I don't. It helps me to indulge those feelings for a little while, maybe by losing sleep or eating a whole pint of ice cream. When I restrict myself from behaving like I feel bad, I also cut myself off from my own ability to process my emotions. In my humble opinion, it's not a sign of strength to stuff down sadness like you never feel it. It's a sign of strength to feel sadness, experience it, and still be able to move on to joy and optimism.

This is probably why that *Rise of the Guardians* scene makes me cry. I *do* believe in monsters, if what that means is there are things about life that will make me sad, hurt, frustrated, angry, disappointed, etc. I'm just not afraid of those feelings, and I know I am strong enough to have those feelings without letting them steal my ability to be happy again.

You, however, are not me, and there may be something else that works for you when you are grieving. The one thing I encourage is for you not to ignore your own emotional needs. Doing so could take more of a toll than you realize on your mind and your body, and that could make it more difficult for you to continue your treatments. You have learn how to be whole now if you want to be whole later, so figure out what that means for you.

4. Get hooked up with a therapist before you need one.

I'm not a psychiatrist, a psychologist, or a doctor of any kind, so I can't tell you what the science is on dealing with grief. Everything I write here is only what has helped me. If you need a few good resources, I've listed some I like in Appendix C at the back of the book.

You know who would have even more reliable resources and research on grief, though? A great therapist. I highly recommend finding one at the beginning of your infertility journey, ideally before you think you need one.

You do not need to be clinically depressed or anxious or have any other big mental health issue to find someone to talk to. Therapists are great for general stress-management. If you don't want to find an individual therapist, a lot of fertility clinics offer free group sessions where you can vent with other people going through the same journey.

Also, that would be a great place to go if you think maybe you'd like a therapist and you have no idea where to find one. But start going early, before the pain hits you. It's much better to have a resource like that on call when you need it than to be scrambling to find one the day you realize you're falling apart.

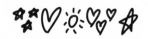

FINAL THOUGHTS ON REPEATED LOSS

You're not a text-book infertility case. You're a real person with unique needs and wants. Give yourself some grace as you go through what will sometimes feel like an absolutely miserable journey. Definitely ignore anyone who makes you feel like they somehow know more about your grief than you do. You know you.

But if you know you are a very strong person normally, and you normally see yourself as someone who barely feels pain, don't expect that to hold true now. Most people can't snowplow through every infertility-related loss without ever experiencing a bad feeling. It would be weirdly un-human to be able to push through everything in a journey like this without any negative repercussions. So be nice to yourself. You're going through something hard. You at least deserve to have *you* on your side!

CHAPTER THIRTEEN
Miscarried Dreams

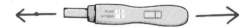

UNFORGIVABLE

It is February 2015, and we have just gotten the best news ever. Our fresh IVF cycle worked! I'm pregnant! I almost can't believe it. I've been going through this for what feels like so long, and finally, finally, we've reached the ultimate goal. I'm going to have a baby.

I am so excited, I completely miss a small detail when the doctor calls to tell us the news. A pregnancy test measures the level of HCG in your body, a hormone that is produced when you're pregnant. A woman is not considered pregnant if her HCG level is below 5 mIU/mL. If your HCG level is anything above 25 mIU/mL, you're considered pregnant. The area between 5 and 25 is a gray area that requires a second test to confirm.[45]

My HCG level is 26 mIU/mL. The doctor tells us that I will need to come back in for a second test in two days and they will be looking for that number to double. I do not read any negativity in his voice at that. Malcolm does. He thinks the doctor is saying, "you're pregnant, *but*."

This causes heaps of trouble for us.

I want to sit in the room we've reserved for the baby's nursery and think about how excited I am. I want to go to all the baby stores and purchase things for the baby. I want to tell our parents immediately, and then I want to share the good news with all my friends who knew I was going through IVF. I am thrilled. I want to celebrate!

Malcolm is reluctant to celebrate. We go to a baby store, and he seems incredibly uncomfortable. We end up not buying anything. He doesn't want to tell his parents, and when he finally does call to tell them, I feel like he's confessing an unplanned pregnancy. It makes me feel ashamed of something I never expected to feel ashamed of.

We've only lived in Georgia for a little over a year, and that move was difficult for us. There was a lot of fighting, mostly because Malcolm refused to take any time off between jobs and I was left to do all of the packing and supervising of movers on my own. We missed a big birthday party for his mother because it happened to fall right when we were moving, and Malcolm seemed to think I was being irresponsible for wanting him to take a *tiny* break and prioritize his family for a minute.

Do you know that scene in the musical *Hamilton* where Eliza begs Alexander Hamilton to take a break? That was me with Malcolm during our move. I felt he was risking major burn out, but actually, what he was putting at risk was our marriage. Something always gives when you fail to take good enough care of yourself. Malcolm did great in the new job, but he and I had terrible fights the year we moved because we were both under so much stress.

Plus, infertility.

So now we're finally pregnant, and my husband doesn't want to celebrate or buy baby clothes or tell his parents, and I'm wondering what the hell I missed. Did Malcolm not want kids after all? Did his parents secretly want our IVF cycle to fail? Is it because they don't like me? Why won't any of them get excited about this baby? I'd thought we'd gotten over most of our post-move fighting. Did I somehow *pressure* Malcolm into this?

My family is as excited as I am, so what's happening here causes strain between our families, too. Then to make it all more complicated, both our sets of parents are visiting this spring, and there's some overlap. My parents are overjoyed, while Malcolm is still acting like he doesn't even want to think about this. His parents barely mention the baby to me at all. When his mother tries to talk to me alone about it—probably meaning to empathize with me and without knowing that Malcolm and I are not on the same page with this—she inadvertently says something that makes me feel like she's telling me I'm not pregnant. She says she had a doctor who told her, "it isn't a baby until the heart beats."

That doctor should be ashamed of himself. That is an awful thing to tell any pregnant woman. Also, we haven't gotten to hear the heartbeat yet, and remember, too, that pregnancy messes with your emotions. I am so bewildered that I think Malcolm's mom is trying to use this story to explain to me why they aren't celebrating. It must be that they don't think this is a true pregnancy, and they feel I shouldn't believe it is either. No one should be excited. This isn't real.

This doesn't go over well with me. By the time Malcolm's parents leave, I'm completely convinced that Malcolm doesn't want the baby and neither do his parents. That has to be it, right? Otherwise, why are they all trying to ignore the fact that I'm pregnant? Why aren't they conveying *any* happiness? Why didn't anyone say *congratulations*?

Now, the baby I wanted so badly before feels like a curse, not a blessing. Then weird things start happening. Symptoms I'd noticed in the beginning—sore breasts and a tiny bit of nausea—disappear. I become extra anxious and upset, and Malcolm and I have one of our worst fights ever. I accuse him of not wanting the baby. I have no memory at all of what he says, but whatever it is does not make me think I've misunderstood his disinterest.

At some point after that fight, I shut myself in our walk-in closet and sit there sobbing. Malcolm doesn't want me to be pregnant, and I don't think he wants me anymore, either. Our marriage is over, and I'm pregnant with a baby my soon-to-be-ex-husband doesn't want, and I've gone through this whole nightmare oblivious to his feelings, so clearly I'm also a terrible wife. This was all an awful mistake.

In a moment of total panic and despair, I pray to God to take the baby away.

I tell God I'll never make this mistake again. I will never, ever try to have a baby with my husband again. I'll leave him. I'll find a different life. If only God will do whatever He needs to do to make this nightmare go away.

I regret that immediately, obviously.

I take it back. I tell God I didn't mean it. I can't imagine giving up that baby, even if it is going to lead to a divorce. I know I've really done it now, though. Because now it's not just my husband who doesn't want me to have the baby. Now *God* is going to punish me for not appreciating the life He created to begin with. I've committed the most appalling sin possible. I regretted getting pregnant.

I try to forget all of that, but around week seven, I go in for the ultrasound they do to find the baby's heartbeat for the first time. There is no heartbeat. The baby is dead.

I have a dilation and curettage (D&C) procedure the next day to remove the tissue. I do not later remember the procedure. I do not remember the day at all. Trauma and anesthesia will do that to you.

Something unexpected happens, though.

Malcolm is just as sad as I am.

As it turned out, he *did* want that baby. His parents wanted us to have the baby. But there was this thing happening that he was able to recognize and I couldn't. Every time the doctors called, Malcolm thought they sounded more dismal about the news. To his ears, the doctors were warning us that the baby wasn't going to survive from the start.

Malcolm was never able to be excited because he never believed the baby had a chance. He'd told his parents the same. So for Malcolm and his parents, the idea of celebrating a baby that wasn't going to live simply wasn't palatable.

This helps me understand what was happening with all of them, but it still takes me a while to forgive Malcolm for not letting me have any hope. I *had* been pregnant. There had been a chance. There was no reason for me to feel any shame about what was going on.

I spend the next several months in a deep depression. I don't ever remember wanting to die, per se, but I do remember fantasizing about the relief suicide could bring. Usually, I can transform that fantasy into a fantasy of taking a very long nap. Ten years of sleep would be good. I'd like to skip forward or backward to some better place.

During this time, I am not on any depression medication. Before I started infertility treatments, my reproductive endocrinologist had advised that I stop my depression medication. Probably I looked fine to him in the office at the time. He doesn't know I have a history of depression, and I do tend to look fine when I'm getting proper help for my depression. It is hard for people who aren't depressed to understand that medication and therapy don't always permanently cure depression. Looking fine doesn't mean you should go off your meds.

But I had stopped the depression meds I'd been on cold-turkey after the doctor advised me to, and I never found a new psychiatrist to help me with that transition. I didn't think I needed one.

This created a problem for me months before we started IVF. It created a problem for me and Malcolm. When our timed intercourse and IUI cycles didn't work in 2014, we both became sad. Malcolm reacted by buying a 1978 Triumph Spitfire for a few thousand dollars. The Spitfire is a sardine can fitted over the body of a go-kart. It doesn't seem to have a functioning top. The seat belts are questionable. There are no airbags. The radio sort of works, but not really.

While he spent his time fixing that car up, I sank into depression. It was so bad in fall of 2014, that every time I rode in that car, I felt I was risking my life, and I really didn't care. I knew that if we even got rear-ended at a stoplight, the car could just squash up around us and kill us, but at the time, the only thing that ever made me feel good was sitting in the passenger seat of the Spitfire, looking up at the sky through an autumn canopy of trees, feeling the wind in my face while Malcolm drove. For my birthday in 2014, Malcolm had brought home a $10 audio cord so I could plug my phone into the Spitfire's radio, play music even when the car antennae wouldn't pick up any radio stations, and sing along. It was the best gift he'd given me in years, but I was still in a dark time.

And that was before the miscarriage. Now we're in an even darker time, my depression is heavier than it's ever been, I'm not on any medication, and the last time I saw a psychiatrist or a therapist, I was living in Chicago. I need serious help, and I don't have any.

If you have never tried to find a good therapist or psychiatrist, you may not know this, but it's quite difficult to do. Turns out, health insurance gets real tricky with mental health professionals, so when you go to find someone, you're likely to discover that half of the mental health professionals in your area are out of network. Of the ones who are in-network, many will ask you to pay them directly and then submit bills to your health insurance. Also, not all of them will be taking new patients, and if they are, they might not have availability for two weeks.

This is why you should get hooked up with at least a therapist *before* you start infertility treatments. If you are prone to depression or anxiety and thinking of going off your medications before you start, you need to make sure you have a mental health provider to help you do that. Because after you've landed in a pit of despair like the one I reached in 2015, finding fresh help can seem near impossible.

I manage to ask my primary care physician to put me back on the same dose of Wellbutrin that I was on before I started IVF. It takes the Wellbutrin a few weeks to kick in, and in the meanwhile, I barely have the energy to do anything. I pull off my work gigs, but otherwise, I sleep all the time, I sit around in the dark with the curtains closed, I binge eat.

I do not know if my marriage is going to survive because Malcolm is sad, too, but he does not understand depression.

He's never had it. He doesn't see why I can't just snap out of it.

I spend time writing. It's easier for me to exist in a fictional fantasy world with characters I create than to exist in the real world. No matter what trouble I give those characters, it's nothing compared to what I'm going through.

The Wellbutrin starts to help. My work schedule gets busy, and that distraction helps, too. I end up in Italy for a work gig in fall of 2015, and Malcolm joins me after the job is over. This gives us a real vacation together, and his phone dies early in the trip, so we get the break we needed. Eventually, I feel better.

Nevertheless, I don't have it in me to try another infertility treatment until 2017. That's how long it takes for me to vanquish my despair entirely. That's how long it takes before I am confident that Malcolm absolutely definitely without a doubt wants kids as much as I do.

I am able to forgive him for everything that happened long before then.

Honestly, though? I'm not sure I'll ever forgive myself. For being so hopeful and naïve about that pregnancy that I didn't understand it was likely to end in miscarriage. For allowing anyone to take away my hope, however slim it should have been. For not understanding what my husband was going through at that time. For bringing our parents into a massive misunderstanding between me and my spouse.

For that one horrible prayer. For miscarrying the baby. I don't think I'll ever be able to convince myself that it wasn't my fault.

I have never before told anyone that entire story.

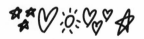

FREQUENTLY ASKED QUESTION

I just had a miscarriage. Will this ever hurt less? How do I get over this? How do I get through this?

ANSWER : ONE MINUTE AT A TIME

This is it. The worst part. There are so many things that hurt about infertility. There's the indignity of it all and all the waiting. There's the toll those drugs take on your body and the feeling that your whole life is being held hostage to unpredictable infertility treatment cycles. There's all the little losses along the way.

But miscarriage is by far the deepest, darkest tragedy of infertility. Or at least it has been for me. When you try and try and try to get pregnant, only to finally get that positive pregnancy result and then have the baby whisked away from you later, it's like getting sucker-punched. Hard.

Then, to pour salt in that wound, you usually can't just try again immediately after. Your body has to recover from a miscarriage with at least one menstrual cycle. Let's suppose you started a fresh IVF cycle at the beginning of January. Then it was the end of February before you found out you were pregnant. Then you miscarried four weeks later at the end of March. You can't just start again in April. You have to wait for your body to finish bleeding out the remnants of the pregnancy. You will then need to wait at least until your next period before you can start another treatment cycle of any kind. If you're lucky, that will be May.

So not only do you have to deal with the emotional blow

of miscarriage, but when it comes to something like IVF, all the things that already hurt about infertility get amplified in the wake of a miscarriage. You need more patience. You deal with more hormones. Your body takes a harder hit. You have to wait and wait and wait.

Miscarriages have range, too. If you're "lucky," you'll have a "missed" miscarriage, meaning that your body will miss that the baby has died for a while. Hopefully, your fertility clinic will notice before your body starts attempting to expel the baby, tissue, and blood you no longer need. If this happens, you'll have options. You could wait for nature to take its course and bleed out the pregnancy whenever your body wants. You could take medication to speed things up. Or you could have a dilation and curettage (D&C), which is a procedure where your doctor will put you under and then surgically remove most of what your body would otherwise have expelled.[46]

Sometimes miscarriage is far more dramatic. I've only had missed miscarriages and D&Cs. I've never had one with television-style miscarriage bleeding, but I know people who have bled a lot with miscarriage. Excessive bleeding is always scary.

Regardless of how your miscarriage happens, your body will have gone through a pregnancy before it occurs. That means no matter how your body gets rid of the pregnancy, it will happen after pregnancy hormones hit your body. You will already have been dealing with things like fatigue and nausea before the miscarriage. This will not make your miscarriage more pleasant.

Miscarriage is hard to get over. I can sympathize with women who've had to do IVF cycle after IVF cycle to get pregnant. I *am* one of those women. I know what that's like.

But my heart truly hurts for women who suffer miscarriage after miscarriage. I've had two. I felt those two were bad enough. I can't imagine how it must hurt to have three, four, five, six miscarriages.

The other rotten thing about miscarriage is how it's still kind of taboo to talk about it. I'm not sure why this is. You're allowed to talk if you have cancer or migraine headaches. If you fall and hurt your back or get injured in a car accident, you can talk about that. If someone you care about dies, you can talk about that.

But if a baby you're carrying dies? No one wants you to talk about that. That's supposed to be private pain.

So women don't talk about it, and that's even though miscarriage is incredibly common. It is estimated that 1 in 4 "recognized" pregnancies end in miscarriage, which usually happens in the first trimester.[47] Since most women don't know they're pregnant until they miss their period, it's also likely that many more pregnancies end in a miscarriage than we know, but we can't count those in the statistics because those women never know they're pregnant.

I suppose maybe the secrecy behind miscarriage is partly because it most often happens in the first trimester, before anyone can see that you're pregnant, and it tends to happen quietly. No one has to know you've gone through it because no one can see it on your body. A massive number of women go through this pain every year and then have to grieve it silently.

But you're not alone if you've miscarried a baby. You're not even alone if you've miscarried a baby and you feel shame related to the miscarriage. It's so easy to feel shame along with losing a baby, and that shame can come from a huge variety of sources. Maybe you had an experience similar to mine, and you feel something you did caused you to lose the baby. Maybe your pregnancy was unplanned and unwanted, and your shame has more to do with the feelings of relief that came with your miscarriage. Maybe your shame is totally irrational. It could just be "my body failed me and killed my baby" shame that you *know* you shouldn't feel but that you feel anyway.

The best thing anyone ever said to me after a miscarriage was, "there was nothing you did to cause this and nothing you could have done to prevent this." That might be the most important thing any woman can understand about miscarriage. The vast majority of the time, you did nothing to kill your baby. This wasn't your fault.

Miscarriage happens for all kinds of reasons, but things like sex, stress, working, exercising, and lifting heavy things aren't on that list.[48] Neither is something you thought or said to God or your mom or your husband or anyone else. We don't always know why a miscarriage occurred. As with all things related to baby-making, miscarriage is not predictable, and it's usually not preventable either. But it wasn't you. You didn't do this.

Yet here we all are, feeling shame over something awful that happened to us—that happened *in* us—and for no good reason at all.

If there's one thing I could say to someone trying to recover from a miscarriage, that's it. **Nothing you did caused your miscarriage, and there was nothing you could have done to prevent it.** Sometimes, life just isn't fair. This bad thing happened *to* you, not *because* of you, and however you're feeling in this moment, the one thing you shouldn't be feeling is self-blame.

Also, there are a million ways to grieve something like

this, and none of them are wrong. You'll need time to get over it. It won't happen overnight. It will hurt.

Some people do things to commemorate babies they've lost in miscarriages. They make memorial jewelry, gardens, and quilts. They order plaques, crystals, signs, teddy bears, and figurines of angels. They donate to charities, name stars, post things on social media every time a miscarriage anniversary passes.

I've never done any of that. Maybe this is because I've had so many other losses, too. We've had two miscarriages, but we've lost at least seven embryos. That's a lot of loss. If I memorialized every embryo, I'd end up with a concrete angel garden that looks a lot like a cemetery.

I keep meaning to put ultrasound pictures in this "adventure book" I started for me and Malcolm before we began infertility treatments. The adventure book was inspired by that Disney movie, *Up*. I gave it to Malcolm on our first anniversary, before we knew infertility would be this hard on us.

Periodically, I go back and watch the opening scene of *Up*. The story is about an old man, but it begins when he is young with a montage of how he met his wife and what they dreamed about for their life together. In the montage, the man meets his wife, they plan to have a home and babies and grand adventures, but then they can't have babies and she gets sick and dies long before he does. They never have the adventure together that they were supposed to have.

There are only a few shots in that montage showing the woman learning she can't have babies, and yet, I've never seen any movie or television show depict infertility so accurately. Disney nailed that sadness. Also, I cry every time I watch that montage. Animation. It gets to me.

But in any case, our adventure book was also supposed

to have a page for every adventure we took, and certainly, a baby is a great adventure, even if you lose that baby. Yet, I haven't touched the adventure book since we made our first appointment with a fertility clinic. I always thought I could update the book after I finally had a baby. So the book has been collecting dust in a box for eight and a half years. Because of this, I guess I can't say too much about whether it is helpful to commemorate miscarriage with memorials of any kind. I avoid commemoration.

Still, there are things I've learned about managing the depression and despair of miscarriage. I went through a hell of a time after my first miscarriage. My second miscarriage, however, was objectively the more tragic miscarriage. It happened later in my first trimester and after several miscarriage scares. We had higher hopes and had already gone through so much. But the grief of that second miscarriage was something I handled far better, partially because Malcolm and I went through it together and partially because I had better personal coping skills.

So here's what I recommend for handling this, the worst part of infertility. These are additions to the recommendations I gave in Chapter Twelve, which are relevant for handling any aspect of infertility grief. But this is what I think applies directly to miscarriage.

INFERTILITY LESSON #14

1. Let yourself grieve.

You just experienced a devastating loss. Therefore, it is normal if you cry, feel sad or hopeless, think the world seems less colorful, lose your appetite or eat too much, are unable to enjoy things you normally enjoy, etc. The abnormal thing would be not to react at all. A little depression after a miscarriage isn't you losing it. It's you going through it.

2. If a reasonable amount of time passes and your grief is interfering with your life, you need to get real help.

There's a line between normal grief and clinical depression, and it's hard to know when you've crossed it. If you don't feel like showering for a couple of days after a miscarriage, that's probably normal grief. If, for a few weeks, you choke up sporadically, binge a few pints of chocolate ice cream or lose some pounds, don't have the attention span for a chick flick, and weep at the sight of the baby clothes you purchased for the baby you just lost, that's probably normal grief, too.

However, if these things happen for long enough that additional bad things occur because of it—like you get in hot water at work for not being able to do your job or you find yourself drinking and driving or your friends feel they need to stage a serious intervention—then you may have crossed into real depression. There's no hard time limit on when this might happen, but if it does happen, it will be much harder for you to fix on your own, and you probably won't be able to just "snap out of it."

If you *can* "snap out of it," then you probably weren't dealing with real depression. In my experience, that's one of the ways you know if you're truly depressed or just grieving and in a bad mood. Someone who is clinically depressed typically cannot simply choose to perk up. Additionally, when you tell them to, they inevitably think about how they can't and what that says about them, and so your attempt to encourage them only confirms for them what an utter failure they are.

A depressed person doesn't want to hurt so bad emotionally that they feel it as physical pain. They don't want to be useless or fatigued. They don't mean to be throwing themselves a pity party. They want to be normal. They just can't figure out how to get there. Something in their brain is blocking the path.

True clinical depression involves a cycle of thoughts, behaviors, and emotions that prevent the depressed person from being able to swim up above the surface and take a breath. It's complex and not easy to solve.[49] If you're there, you likely need professional help, which could include therapy or depression medications.

Don't delay getting that help if you think you might need it. Start looking around for someone *as soon* as you realize you're in trouble. Then, once you find a mental health professional, let that professional help you.

Avoid assuming that once you're "better," you no longer need help, especially if you are continuing your infertility treatments. I have stayed on Wellbutrin since I went back on it after my miscarriage in 2015. This is something I've discussed with my reproductive endocrinologists and my psychiatrists. For me, it is far better to take a medication for my depression than to spend months unable to enjoy anything, binge eating on a couch in the dark, and thinking suicidal thoughts about how worthless I am as a person. When I'm behaving like that, I know it's not me. It's the depression, and I see no reason to live like that.

I also continue to see a therapist, and no, I don't think either the meds or the therapy make me a different or less capable person. I think the opposite. The help I get from drugs and therapy prevents a physiological illness from taking over my brain and body and blocking my ability to stay healthy. As far as I'm concerned, anyone who judges me for seeking and accepting that help can go to hell. Or possibly they're already in hell. After all, no one gets points for refusing depression meds or therapy, but they do suffer needlessly. There's no reason for that to be me or you.

3. Be kind to your partner.

You and your partner may not feel or react to a miscarriage the same way. You might need more or less time to cope. You might need different tools. You might need to cry more or less. You might need to laugh more or less. All that is fine.

No matter what differences you have, though, the one thing you probably have in common is how much you need each other right now. So this is not the moment to withdraw from your relationship. This is the moment to cling to it, to take cover in it, and to take comfort in the fact that you're riding this out together. There's something about sharing pain that lessens it overall, so be a little extra kind and loving with your partner right now, and accept extra hugs and kisses while you both deal with this. Don't do this alone.

4. Whatever you need to recover is okay.

You're not me. You're not your friend who's had six miscarriages and always seems fine right after. You're not your family member who has never had a miscarriage and thinks you're taking too much time to grieve or not enough. You're not that woman on Pinterest who has the beautiful miscarriage memorial garden that seems to be the place where she plants her grief. You're not the woman in the novel who cracks and becomes a paranoid baby stealer after one miscarriage.

You're you, and you're dealing with *your* pain and loss. Don't let anyone tell you that you're doing grief wrong. In fact, don't judge your grief at all. You have enough on your plate with this already, don't you? Your only job with your miscarriage grief is to process it as well as you can so that you can keep living your life and trying again with another fertility cycle if that's what you want.

So look for the color in life again when you can. Try for another baby if you want. Stop trying if you can't withstand any more. Get help if you need it. Take it easy on yourself and your partner. Miscarriage is a destroyer. Give yourself what you need to recover from that.

FINAL THOUGHTS ABOUT MISCARRIAGE

As I said in the previous chapter, I'm not a psychiatrist, a psychologist, or a doctor of any kind, and I have no expertise with fixing grief except for what has helped me with my own. However, check out Appendix C for more resources at the back of the book. The resource that helped me the most with my grief was Megan Divine's book, *It's Okay that You're Not Okay*. If you're feeling shame, I recommend looking into Brené Brown's work on shame and vulnerability. If you're trying not to feel this at all, you might pick up *The Body Keeps the Score* by Bessel Van der Kolk MD.

My second miscarriage was far more devastating than my first. But by the time I went through it, Malcolm and I were both so much better at grief and coping that we rode it out fairly well. I did feel a lot of sadness over that miscarriage—I still feel that sadness sometimes—but I never experienced any shame about it. I'm even kind of proud of us both for having learned how to fall apart without completely falling apart. I've written more about that in Chapter Fifteen, a chapter about ways infertility can make you stronger.

And there are lots of good things about infertility. So now, let's talk about the silver linings. Not everything that happens to you on an infertility journey is for the worst. There are blessings, too. Miscarriage just isn't one of them.

PART V
Perspective

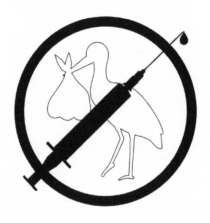

The circumstances we ask God to
change are often the circumstances
God is using to change us.
~ Mark Batterson

CHAPTER FOURTEEN
Don't Be a Diva

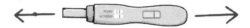

FREQUENTLY ASKED QUESTION

I am so incredibly stressed about my infertility treatments! I feel like I can barely breathe when I think about everything I've gone through. I spend all my time crying on the bathroom floor because this is just so awful. I'm so lost. What I am going through is worse than what anyone else has ever gone through. When I am not crying, I spend my time posting on social media about what a wreck I am, and—

ANSWER: STOP. PLEASE.

I know this hurts.

In so many ways.

This is exhausting, stressful, disappointing, outrageous, depressing, anxiety-provoking, patience-testing, infuriating, devastating, etc., etc.

Your hormones are all over the place. Your body is held hostage by your desire and inability to produce children. Your life is on stand-still. Sometimes, you don't know if you'll ever feel hopeful again, and sometimes, you feel freakishly hopeful, and sometimes, you have no idea how you feel.

Additionally, you Googled this, so you happen to know that infertility is just as stressful as cancer.[50] I bet you feel like your infertility is even *worse* than cancer. Cancer patients at least get to talk openly about chemo and walk in fundraising events for survivors. Where's your damn parade? You're suffering, and you have no idea when it will end, and oh, yeah, you're also depressed and anxious and experiencing psychosomatic symptoms of infertility like migraine headaches and hives and IBS.

So yes, I get it. You're in a bad place.

Now, grab some tissues, blow your nose, wipe off the mascara you smeared all over your face while you were crying on the bathroom floor, get yourself a glass of ice water or a cup of hot tea, do not go anywhere *near* any of your social media accounts, and pull yourself together.

Because I know this is bad, but it is not your diva pass.

Ouch. That sounded mean and insensitive. You may have tried to block it out. Perhaps I should repeat it.

Infertility is not your excuse to be a dramatic, woe-is-me, triggered-by-everything diva.

Confession: my husband has never allowed me to diva-out over infertility, and sometimes, that has made me furious at him. Enraged furious. Red-hot furious. "I deserve to be sensitive, difficult, and witchy right now!" furious. I mean, come on! There are a million movies about crazy-hormonal pregnant women freaking out over inconsequential things. In the movies, the woman is always allowed to collapse to the kitchen floor crying. Then her spouse or partner sits down next to her, and a heartwarming, adorable bonding scene ensues.

My husband, who strongly dislikes being wrong or told what to do, is far more likely to react to me being overly-sensitive by snapping back, getting angry at me, or just plain ignoring me. The phrase, "Stop throwing yourself a Sandy Pity Party" was used in my house so many times one year when we were doing IVF treatments that I truly hated the term "pity party."

There have been a couple of times when Malcolm genuinely screwed up this way. I've already mentioned that he had a very difficult time understanding when I was depressed. He would say, "Why can't you just be happy?" and I would think, "I would be happy if I could be happy, but I can't be happy, and you clearly think this is a fundamental flaw in my personality, and obviously I am failing at life, omg, I want to die."

If I haven't said it before, a clinically depressed person can't "just be happy." That's exactly their problem. They would be happy if they had that choice. They'd gratitude-pep-talk their way to happiness in a heartbeat if that was an option. It's not, though, so let's carve out an exception to the rule in this chapter. **If you can't get yourself up from the bathroom floor, and if my initial advice about that makes you feel like a total failure, and if you feel that you're about to spiral down into a worse depression than you were already in, then this chapter doesn't apply to you.** Refer back to Chapter Thirteen and get help. Do not read any further here.

But for the rest of you—and please be honest with yourself here as to where you really fall—as much as I would have liked for my husband to indulge my "pity parties" from time to time, I mostly think that when Malcolm refused to be a guest at a Sandy Pity Party, he was right not to show up.

Now, there are times when the stress and hormones of infertility can turn an otherwise calm person into an irritable monster. Partners, sometimes you need to back off when your wife or girlfriend is two weeks into an estrogen binge that's got her feeling like she should be screaming or crying all the time.

Let me put this into plain words. If you observe the woman you love shrieking bloody murder at you because you used the wrong pan to cook the lasagna in, and she is in the middle of an IVF cycle, and this is not normal, then I don't care what kind of day you're having. Please just set down the pan, hand her some ice cream, and say, "I know this is hard." Then step away. Or at least don't take it personally. This is not you. This is her having a lousy hormone day. Don't ask me how I know.

That being said, if you are going through infertility struggles, you should not be sitting around regularly, telling yourself how bad it is, day after day after day. That won't help you. If anything, it will only train you to believe that you actually *do* have it really bad. That pattern of repetitive negative thoughts can harm your brain.[51] You don't want to do that to yourself.

The truth is, as much as infertility sucks, and as much as I appreciate that we all need to vent sometimes, your infertility is unlikely to be an epic tragedy full of so much despair that no one else has ever experienced this kind of despair before.

So here's what I want to say if you are reading this book because you want someone to validate your desire to wallow in your misery:

Get over yourself.

This is also worth repeating. Attention super special snowflakes, personal justice warriors, social media drama hogs, trigger-trend seekers: you aren't the first person in human history to struggle with having children. Not even close.

Humans have been fighting infertility for at least as long as the collective human memory exists. The first infertility story of the Bible happens in Genesis, chapters 15-21. To Abraham and Sarah. Abraham. You know, the "father of many?" The first patriarch of the Jewish people?

The only stories that come before Abraham's story are: (1) God creates the world from nothing; (2) God creates man from dust (Adam); (3) God creates woman from man (Eve); (4) humans fall from grace/sin (Eve eats an apple, offers it to Adam, and is forever cursed with painful childbirth); (5) the first murder (Cain kills Abel); (6) the first natural disaster (Noah and the flood); (7) humans begin to speak more than one language (Tower of Babel). Then we get to (8) a man screws up in every way and struggles with infertility, but eventually he has enough faith that God gives him a son and makes him the father of, like, everything. That's Abraham.

After, Genesis is all a lot of family drama, sex, affairs, betrayal, prosperity, famine, prophecy, and death. Then the Israelites get stuck in Egypt, away from the promised land, cue Exodus, Moses, and a bunch of plagues that weren't quite as bad as what happened to all of us in 2020.

That was "Genesis in a Nutshell: A Story of Sex, Babies, and Disasters" by Sandy Vasher, a Christian feminist who actually does believe in God.

Anyway. In the very first book of a very old sacred scripture that millions of people today still base their religious beliefs on, infertility only comes after three other problems: sin, murder, and natural disaster. *That's* how relevant infertility has been to the collective human experience. It's after sin, murder, and the flood, but before everything else.

So no. Your inability to have children is nothing someone else hasn't gone through before. Your fight isn't new. Your feelings aren't fresh. *You* may be discovering this for the first time, but that doesn't mean this problem hasn't previously existed. Infertility has been around forever.

Obviously, the fact that we as a species have cared so much about our ability to procreate for so long means that infertility is legitimately disruptive. You certainly deserve to feel deep pain and grief over this. You will have hard days because of this. You will be socially isolated, your body will feel physical distress. You are allowed to cry. It is incredibly human to feel that you are being denied some basic, essential part of life when you can't have children. I don't want you to pretend that's not happening to you.

But at the same time, you shouldn't make this struggle your own personal misery membership. It's not personal. It's common. According to the Centers for Disease Prevention and Control, 6% of married women age 15-44 have trouble getting pregnant after one year of trying.[52] You're not alone here. You're experiencing something plenty of other people have experienced before and gotten through.

So, you can throw yourself a couple of pity parties here and there, but you need to phase those out over time the same way mature adults phase out massive birthday parties as they get older. At some point, celebrating your own misery just isn't good for you anymore. Acknowledging, feeling, and processing pain is one thing. But swimming in it like it's chocolate syrup you want to be drowning in is self-indulgent and likely to make you feel worse. Wallowing only feels good for a limited amount of time. Then you need to get out of your chocolate syrup and wash up.

When I'm having a hard time pulling myself out, I find it useful to remind myself that *because* the pain of infertility is such a universal, across-space-and-time kind of thing, I don't get to act like I got dealt a particularly bad hand in life. Infertility has been hard on me, and I've struggled because of it. But *everyone* struggles. *Life* is a struggle. We all go through things that hurt, and often, we face that hurt silently and alone. Maybe infertility is my current hurt, but my friend who has what seems to be the perfect family, kids, dog, car, home, etc., could be going through something else that hurts just as much. I might not even know about it.

This is a good time to talk about privilege and infertility, too. Malcolm and I both have all kinds of things going for us. We're white, straight, cisgender, and well-educated. We are healthy and financially secure.

Our parents are all four healthy and financially secure, and both sets of our parents are still married. We grew up in safe, comfortable homes. Neither of us has ever been abused. We've never gone hungry. We've never been homeless. We were raised to be resilient and given great opportunities. We've taken fabulous vacations, we have expensive tastes in wine. Hell, our *og* is a little white privileged dog.

We weren't handed everything. My husband and I were both focused students when we were younger, we accumulated a lot of educational debt, and we work very hard now. We are not rich. We are not independently wealthy. We have to continue to work to sustain our privileged lifestyle. But we also know we started off incredibly lucky and blessed.

Our lives are not a tragedy.

To me, it's important to keep that perspective in mind, because in many ways, Malcolm and I have been lucky just to be on the infertility journey we've taken. A lot of couples wouldn't be able to sustain eight years of this. Infertility treatments are only rarely covered by health insurance, and even when they are covered, it's not usually complete coverage.

We've had pretty good health insurance throughout the years, but the vast majority of our infertility treatments were not covered by insurance. Appendix B is a chronology of our infertility treatments and what we paid for those treatments from 2011 to 2020. When I tally up what we've spent, I come to a total of $64,866. That's out-of-pocket cash, not what an insurance company paid, and it's probably a low estimate because I didn't save every receipt.

On average, a fresh IVF cycle costs anywhere from $12,000 to $17,000 in the U.S., not including medication, which could cost a few thousand more.[53] Add genetic testing, and you are likely to add thousands or so on top of that. So you could be looking at anywhere from $17,000 to $27,000 for a single fresh IVF cycle with whatever bells and whistles you add. We spent about $17,407 on our first fresh cycle, and we didn't do any genetic testing that time. For our second, we spent $24,405, and that did include genetic testing plus more diagnostic testing than the first fresh cycle required.

In our experience, a "frozen" IVF cycle costs more like $4,000 to $6,000. At least one recent study suggests that women are likely to need six IVF cycles to get one live birth, though most couples only do three to four IVF cycles total.[54]

So let's do a little math problem. Suppose you only need one fresh IVF cycle and two frozen cycles—no genetic testing—to have one baby. Let's also suppose that you're at a relatively inexpensive clinic. Finally, let's suppose your

insurance doesn't cover anything except the basics (progesterone shots and estrogen). You could expect to spend the
following:

$12,000 for your first fresh cycle + $3,000 for meds
$4,000 for your first frozen cycle + $250 for meds
$4,000 for your second frozen cycle + $250 for meds
Total: $23,500.

You could buy a decent car for that amount of money. But
who has that just lying around? In 2019, the median American household income was $68,703.[55] So you don't have to be
"underprivileged" to struggle with the costs of infertility. If
you are a normal household, sitting right there in the middle
of American household incomes, the cost of your infertility
cycles could be 34% of your annual household income.

Not only that, but as of August 2020, only 19 states had
laws about fertility insurance coverage, of which only 13
included IVF coverage.[56] So the scenario I laid out is realistic,
except that it doesn't involve the costs of any diagnostic tests
(which are sometimes covered by insurance but will probably still require you to spend some out-of-pocket cash).

It would be realistic not to start with IVF, but timed
intercourse cycles and IUI can be expensive, too. We spent
about $2,000 per cycle on our first timed intercourse cycle
and our two IUI cycles because that was a year when our
insurance didn't cover any infertility treatments. If my math
is right, a normal infertile couple without insurance could
easily spend $30,000 to have a baby.

That's a lot of cash.

The financial costs alone make infertility far easier on
an affluent couple in the U.S. than a poor couple or even an
average couple. But now imagine all the other barriers that
exist for anyone at all underprivileged.

Racial disparity would be the obvious issue to look at next. The disparities that make medical care in the U.S. worse and more expensive for black people than white people apply to infertility as much as any other aspect of health care.[57]

That's just one problem, too. What happens if there's a language barrier between you and your medical provider at a fertility clinic? How easy is it for you to get to a fertility clinic if you work a job with inflexible hours and you don't get many days off? What if you don't have a car? What if you are paid hourly? What if your cultural background makes you less likely to seek medical help to begin with? Or mental health help?

Infertility affects people across race, ethnicity, sexuality, gender, class, and income lines. But if you're not wealthy, white, straight, married, and well-educated, your access to infertility treatments could be limited by all kinds of factors. I speak from my own perspective when I say that even a very privileged person can get tired of this. Anyone could want to give up. If you are also fighting socio-economic barriers, infertility could be too high a mountain to climb.

The way I see this, infertility isn't a privileged-person problem, but it *is* a battle privileged-persons can take on for longer and with more resources than anyone else.

Though life can come with some real surprises no matter who you are, huh? When Covid-19 hit, fertility clinics across the country shut their doors for an unknown amount of time. Some clinics were forced to cancel cycles, even for couples who were mere *days* from an IVF transfer.[58] Infertility treatments, after all, are "elective." It wasn't safe to continue during a pandemic.

Never mind the millions of young, fertile couples who were told to wash their hands, wear masks, and shelter at home, but not to abstain from sex. There will be plenty of Covid-19 babies born in 2020 and 2021, and no one will perceive that as a problem. But thousands of couples were devastated when their fertility cycles were unexpectedly halted thanks to Covid-19.

Malcolm and I were in the middle of an IVF cycle right then ourselves, and our cycle thankfully did not get canceled. Still, I grieve for the couples whose reproductive lives were put on hold thanks to the pandemic. Even six months is a lot of time in the world of infertility, and there were no guarantees for couples who had to cancel cycles. When would they get to start up again? Would they need to redo tests in a year because their body had changed? Would their egg supply diminish in the meanwhile? How would their age affect their chances? No one knew.

And what about the money? Fertility clinics aren't in the business of helping patients out financially. Fertility clinics have to make money, so they're more like casinos when it comes to dollars and cents. You go in to roll the most expensive dice ever, the odds are stacked against you, and the house always wins. So what happened to the couples who were already pinching pennies to pay for an IVF cycle but then lost their jobs during the pandemic? How do those couples start their infertility treatments again? Or does Covid-19 shatter their hopes of having children entirely?

My infertility journey has been long, but if there's one thing I've learned throughout this journey, it's that someone always has it worse. Wherever you fall on the privilege spectrum, that's likely to be true for you, too. It's important to keep your pain in perspective. When you're in the mood to pity yourself, try to keep it in check. This probably isn't as bad as it can get.

INFERTILITY LESSON #15

1. Before you decide that you have it worse than everyone else because of your infertility, take a look around. Keep some perspective. Someone else always has it worse.

2. Before you post something on social media about your infertility, check to make sure you're not swiping a diva pass with your post. Does this post make you seem like you think you're the only person dealing with infertility? Does it make you seem like you think you're the only person dealing with pain? If so, perhaps a revision is in order.

3. Before you throw your next self-pity party, consider canceling. Dry those tears. Pick yourself up from the bathroom floor. Maybe push your party back a little if you still want to host it at some point. But mostly? It's time to phase self-pity out of your life.

4. Before you decide you're a failure for not being able to cancel your pity party, seek help! You may have clinical depression. That's not your fault. Go find a professional who can help you work through it!

5. Before you start infertility treatments, call your insurance company and find out what's covered for you. Most fertility clinics have a finance or billing department that can help you estimate your costs. Ask them to include possible diagnostic tests. Get clear information about your expected costs before you begin a new cycle.

6. Before the next election, check out what your state requires in terms of mandatory insurance coverage for infertility treatments. Now would be a great time to write to your congressional representatives about this.

Plenty of insurance companies cover male sexual dysfunction. If they pay for Viagra, they should be covering IVF. (P.S. Check out Resolve.org for more information on how you can be an advocate for other people facing infertility.)

FINAL THOUGHTS ABOUT INFERTILITY AS A TRAGEDY

Infertility sucks a lot. There are moments when you need to take care of yourself, and some of that means letting yourself feel bad for you. On occasion. But don't let yourself live in self-pity. You have so many better things to do than to feel bad for yourself right now! There is personal growth in every story of struggle, and infertility can be an opportunity for that growth if you let it. Read on to the next chapter to find out more about that. It's time to focus on the positive.

CHAPTER FIFTEEN
Let This Make You Stronger

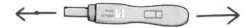

THE INFERTILITY PARADOX

Infertility is the perfect life crisis.

No, I'm not being sarcastic. I was an incredibly anxious child, and I used to spend a lot of time worrying about what horrible things my future might hold. I had an unnatural fear of early death via car accidents, shootings, fires, and plane crashes. The fear lasted into my twenties, and I even thought I had proof that bad things were coming for me. There were a few years when every single time I took a road trip, some scary random thing would happen. Like a mattress falling off the back of a pickup truck right in front of me in a snow storm. It wasn't hard for me to convince myself that a dark cloud was hanging over my head.

Fortunately, three very useful things happened to help me shake that feeling in my thirties. First, a very kind therapist told me no research says getting struck by terrible disasters is tied to any pattern. You could be hit by lightning three times in a row or never hit. We have no evidence supporting the premise that God has everyone's name in a hat and He's drawing names to see whose turn it is to be struck by the next tragedy, disaster, or semi-truck. That's not how this works.

I'm pretty sure that therapist was making the research thing up for my sake. However, she still deserves a medal for helping me come to the realization that you can't control or prevent the randomly bad things that happen in life. And once you come to terms with your inability to control or prevent bad things, it's hard not to feel that you need to live as though every good minute is a gift.

The second thing that happened occurred while my husband and I were on a road trip together. We were in a car he'd had forever, and I started complaining that the passenger airbag light was going off. We were on the interstate, and I saw the light go off again. I opened my mouth to nag Malcolm about that light—because what if we were in an accident and I needed the passenger airbag?—and the rear control arm of our car broke. The car began skidding around.

My airbag didn't go off, and later, we got a look at the control arm. It was snapped in half. But I wasn't hurt, and neither was the rest of the car. Malcolm is a damn good driver, and somehow, he managed to keep the car from slamming into anything after the control arm broke. He even managed to steer it to the side of the road and coast to a nearby exit. We were driving through downtown Louisville, and that exit spat us out right in front of a big hotel. Some guy gave us a "thumbs up" as Malcolm was miraculously preventing his car from killing us. He especially likes that part of the story.

But for me, this was the universe saying something like, "You can't be in charge of how this game of life goes. All you can do is marry a guy who knows how to drive and hope for the best." I think it made me feel like I really ought to stop worrying and start being thankful for the luck I've had so far.

The third thing that happened is infertility.

Which, of course, is where this was all going. There have been a few times when I've thought maybe if God has a deck of disaster cards that He's dealing out, then I got dealt "infertility" as my disaster card. Infertility can be a decent disaster, but if it really is part of the "disaster deck," I now think it's a pretty lucky card.

Here's why: infertility is the kind of disaster that destroys your dreams and life expectations. (Stay with me here.) You thought you were going to have four kids. Nope. You thought you were going to be a mom by twenty-nine. Nope. You thought all the vacations you took in your thirties were going to be kid-friendly vacations to national parks and monuments. Nope.

Instead of all that, you get cut off from your dreams and expectations. Then you put a substantial amount of time, money, and energy into trying to get pregnant.

But it's still a great disaster card. Because despite all the ways infertility interferes in your life, it is not an ax that separates you from everything you ever cared about. Your marriage could go through rough times and your friendships could change. Your career could go down an unexpected and initially unwanted path. Your body could get fatter while your wallet gets thinner.

However, none of that is the same as losing someone you dearly love, becoming terminally ill, or being injured and disabled in a car accident. It's not the same as losing your job or getting divorced because your spouse cheated on you. It's not the same as severe mental illness. The pain of infertility *can* add up over time, but it is not a thunderbolt that strikes you down in an instant and rips away everything you love.

What infertility does more than anything is separate you from a *future* you planned, not a present you are currently living. And as paradoxical as this might sound, about the best thing you can lose is the idealized expectation you had for your future.

Why? Because when you lose something that hasn't happened yet, what you are left with is an enormous world of other, different possibilities that you may never even have thought about before.

Infertility closes the first few doors you thought you were going to walk through in the hallway of life. But once you get a little farther down the hall, you come to the point where you realize there are an *infinite* number of doors in your future, all of which could lead to interesting, amazing, beautiful things in your life and none of which you would have gotten to if you'd taken one of those early doors.

I'm being excessively metaphorical, huh?

Okay, so I'll admit that it took a long time for me to understand that infertility is a part of life that has changed me for the better. There have been plenty of times when I've wallowed in infertility as though it is my life tragedy. I'll also admit that the change infertility forces you through isn't exactly a metamorphosis from caterpillar to butterfly. It's longer than that and more challenging. You don't necessarily see it coming. Change sometimes sneaks up on you, though.

I recently had a conversation with a friend I hadn't spoken to in many years. I rented a room in her apartment while I was in my third year of law school. She was not going to law school and was not a lawyer (which endeared her to me). But she was about ten years older than me, and when I met her, she'd already left a first career to pursue a second career that would give her more freedom. She was dating a genuinely nice guy, she was extroverted, friendly, kind, pretty, adventurous, and most importantly, she knew how to be stressed and happy at the same time.

Summary: she was a role model.

When I moved out of her apartment at the end of the year, I felt I had learned many critical things, like "Drinking pink champagne with your girlfriends is the best" and "Starting a new relationship can be as simple as asking someone you want to get to know better to have lunch with you."

The biggest lesson was that being content with life—being stressed and happy at the same time—has a lot to do with your own attitude, regardless of what's going on around you. You don't need to have it all figured out yet. You don't need to be an all-star achiever. You don't need a million dollars, a Supreme Court clerkship, or a bestselling novel. You only need to be balancing your life well enough that the happiness roughly outweighs the stress.

I made it my goal to learn how to be as balanced as this particular friend by the time I turned thirty. I did not meet that goal. At thirty, I was still *far* from knowing how to be happy even some of the time, and I was very stressed out. I had just quit my job as a high-paid attorney and taken a job as a consultant, but I had no idea where that might take me long-term. I had allowed the leader of a writing group to shatter my confidence, and I was hardly doing any writing at all. I had only just gotten married, and Malcolm and I were having arguments about how many kids we should have. I was nervous and a little depressed, and my struggles with infertility were still on the horizon. I didn't think I'd ever find that "balance" I wanted.

Fast forward eight years, and I'm talking to this same

friend on the phone. To my eyes, she is still the perfect role model. She's happily married to that same nice guy, and they have two great kids. She home schools her kids and runs various groups for them. She organizes a community garden. She's extroverted, friendly, kind, pretty...

I find myself thinking maybe *I* should make it a goal to be running a community garden by the time I'm forty because that's how idealistic this sounds to me.

Then we start talking about my life and she remembers that I wanted to be a writer way back when I was in law school. "And you did it!" she says. "You actually wrote your book! You wouldn't have had time for that if you had kids!" This makes me think of all the other things I've done, too, and it's a lot.

In some ways, this friend of mine is living exactly the life I thought I wanted ten years ago. My dreams of having that life with those kids were dashed by infertility, and oh, the tears I've shed over that. I thought I was wasting so much time with infertility.

Yet, when I start thinking of the life I've lived over the last decade, I realize that the things I've done and accomplished really do outweigh the dreams I wasn't able to fulfill. I'll probably never run a community garden, but I've lived in three states, I have friends all over the country, and I co-run a YouTube channel for writers. Maybe one day, I'll run community writer's workshops or host writer's retreats. The thought of doing that makes me happy, and it's not unrealistic.

I still don't have those kids, but I do have a dog who I love like she's a little, ten-pound princess. I have acquired hobbies I wouldn't have had time for with kids. I quilt, crochet, craft, read, bake. I have been known to attend conferences for liberal feminist Christians, grow orchids and African violets, and enjoy a glass of spicy, bold red wine while taking a bubble bath and reading a book.

The pandemic of 2020 hit, and I looked around at all these people my age who felt like they were going stir-crazy at home with "nothing to do," and I thought, "I don't understand. How can you have *nothing* to do?" My life is full and rich, and I'm never bored because there's always another story to write, another sewing project to complete, another recipe to master, another walk to take with the dog.

Not only that, but I can't imagine these things disappearing from my life if I have kids. That's one of the wildest changes that has happened for me because of infertility. My friends who are moms are very fond of telling me that once I have children, I won't have time for writing or sleeping or any of my hobbies. Life will all be about my kids.

They would probably have been right if I'd had my kids in my early thirties. If that had happened, I'd have been a perfectionistic, Pinterest-oriented parent who worried about grades and achievements and whether my toddler was Ivy-league bound.

Now, any kids I have will be raised during my late thirties and early forties, and I will not be *anything* like the parent I would have been a decade ago. Because now I know it's actually incredibly important for kids to see their parents as whole people.

I want any kids I have to get lots of attention but also to see that mom has goals that don't relate to them. I want them to see me working on my books. I want them to see me getting crazy obsessive over a new do-it-yourself project that isn't for them. I want them to be *bored* sometimes so they can learn how to creatively, independently, and imaginatively entertain themselves. (Because you never know when it might become really important to be able to keep yourself busy.)

Do you think that will make me a bad mom? Guess what? *I do not care what you think.* That's another way infertility has changed me for the better. I no longer live to meet anyone else's expectations about what I should be. I live to pursue the things I'm passionate about and to see what great adventure life might hold for me next. I live to see what things will bring me joy, and I live to see what I can do to make the world a better place (but *not* because I care what *you* think of me).

Oh, and I believe I am capable of doing these things, even when I'm stressed as hell. I'm resilient—far more so than I used to be—and this is also a "gift" of infertility. After all, infertility is the kind of challenge that forces you to develop patience and grit while requiring you to let go of obsession and the need to control and plan your life. To get through this, you *have* to learn how to compartmentalize pain and loss and let hope and happiness win over fear and stress. You have to figure out some legit balance. You have to get stronger. I had to get stronger.

I became who I am today because I had to get over people giving me unsolicited advice, time-after-time, about how to have kids and why I could not give up on those kids. Because I had to get over not having the privacy I thought I'd always have with regard to my own body. Because I had to learn how to cope with my depression and stay positive even when I felt irreparably sad. Because I had to drop my expectations about what a "perfect" life looks like and give up my pre-existing ideals.

Ten years ago, I thought life was about having a couple of kids, being an amazing mom and wife, and pursuing a stable, upward career trajectory. That's not what I think today, and I think I'm better for it. Or at least I think that if you got stuck in an elevator with me for an afternoon, you'd find me a far more interesting person now than I was before this whole ordeal began.

You see what I'm talking about with those doors?

Look, I'd have gladly taken those babies I wanted years before, and I don't think I'd have regretted who they made me. But I don't see the point in looking back at the life you've lived and regretting how it changed you. I *do* see the point in looking back and counting your blessings, your accomplishments, the skills you've developed, and the strength you've gained despite or because of the hard things you've faced. So the way I see it, I'm lucky that I got dealt "infertility." I've lost things, but I gained more than I lost.

If infertility is your current disaster card, then I hope you're starting to experience some of the ways this can make you better. If you're struggling, here are some specific recommendations I have for turning infertility from a trauma into a "self-improvement" exercise.

INFERTILITY LESSON #16

1. Acquire a "gain frame" perspective.

My mother has a PhD in psychology, and her thesis was about positive psychology. Because of this, I have a solid shelf full of self-help books like, "The How of Happiness" by Sonja Lyubomirsky.

Mom, in case you think my shelf of self-help books isn't crowded enough, you should probably know that I pick up all kinds of these books on my own to listen to on Audible or read on my Kindle. I probably listen to or read at least one inspirational, self-help book a month. I keep a gratitude journal. I write down things I'm proud of accomplishing at the end of the month. I give myself pep talks. I get outside when I need to cheer up. I take my happiness seriously.

Having said that, I will also say that I believe happiness is a very personal endeavor that isn't just about keeping your chin up. One person's Saturday morning run is another person's version of hell. One person's snarky-smart-ass attitude is another person's snotty-rude attitude. As far as I can tell, the trick is to figure out what genuinely makes *you* feel good about the world and try to get as much of that in your life as possible.

I am the kind of person who needs to feel sad to feel happy, so I embrace sadness as a healthy emotion, especially as it pertains to infertility loss. But it is one thing to let yourself feel sad, and it's another to constantly look at life in terms of what you don't have. It is hard to reap any positive benefits from a tough situation when you only see what that situation has taken from you.

So here's the thing: you need a gain frame to get the benefits of infertility that I've been talking about. This means you focus not on what you've lost and can't get back but what you've gained or what you could gain. If I think about the babies I've lost, I only feel sad and hopeless. If I think about the books I've published and the businesses I've started, I feel encouraged, proud, and hopeful. If I think about what I've put my body through, I feel discouraged. If I think about the new handbags I have time to sew every year, I feel pleased.

This is the same for my husband. He's had time to focus on his career and work long hours that maybe he wouldn't have wanted to work if we'd had babies at home. He's had weekends to fix up old cars and drive some of those cars out to the mountains where he can fly down curvy roads for as long as he wants. Tough to do that with a toddler around.

We've taken beautiful weekend drives together in those cars, rolling through pretty country roads with the top down and music blasting from staticky old speakers. We've taken very cool kid-unfriendly vacations someone who had to save up for a family trip couldn't afford. We've shipped home a lot of wine. It's easier to do that stuff when you don't have kids.

We used to have a recurring fight where Malcolm would say, "Once we have kids, we'll have to give all this up. Everything will be about our kids." I would argue that giving up everything for your kids is bad parenting.

I don't know if it is or isn't, but I know that I probably won't ever feel that any sacrifice I make for a child is anything but a gain. Maybe we'll have to alter our activities if we have kids. Maybe I'll write children's books instead of romance novels. Maybe my husband will spend less time driving and more time fixing up his cars with a little mechanic by his side. Will we see this as giving anything up? No. We'll view it as adding something to the life we've created. That's our gain perspective at work.

You can do this for yourself. Just ask yourself a simple question: what do you get to do these days that you couldn't have done if you had a baby in your arms right now? And while you're answering the question, try not to compare. I'm sure you'd *rather* have that baby, but that isn't the reality you live in for now. Focus on what you do have that makes you feel happy and fulfilled instead.

Framing infertility as something you gain from will prevent the losses from feeling so overwhelming. Choose to see the positive time after time, and you may be surprised to discover one day that you've even trained yourself to feel pretty good about what you do have. Perspective is everything.

2. Be creative about building your legacy.

I think one of the hardest things to face in infertility is the possibility that you won't leave a legacy behind if you don't have kids.

Have you seen that Disney movie, *Coco*? I loved it (I love animated movies generally, if you can't tell by now), but if I'd watched it at the beginning of my infertility struggle, I might have hated it because the whole story is premised on a Mexican cultural belief that you die twice: once when your physical body dies and the second time when the last living person who remembered your name forgets you.

In the movie, the people who are supposed to remember you after your first death are your family members. But when you face the possibility of never having kids, there's a real chance that you will not have any family that remembers you after you die. That's a hard thing to positive-talk your way out of.

But you can have a legacy regardless of whether you have kids, and this is one of the places where infertility can make you more interesting as a person. You just need to get creative about your legacy. After all, that's what you're missing because of infertility, right? The ability to create something that lives on after you? Well, you don't have to give that up just because you can't have kids. There are so many ways to be remembered that don't involve birthing a baby.

For me, building a legacy means storytelling. Writing books is one way I can leave my mark without having children. I may not end up with grandchildren who will remember me, but I could end up with readers who remember me. That's a legacy that will outlast me.

Does that appeal to you? Are you a creative person in some other way? An artist of another kind? If not, there are plenty of other pathways to make sure your life counts. Find a cause you're passionate about and volunteer for an organization that supports that cause. Be remembered by the people you help. Start a business that reflects something you care deeply about. Be remembered by the people you inspire. The work you do today can touch lives in ways that matter long after you're gone.

If you don't like your work or you don't have a cause or passion, now is your chance to be flexible with your career. Go back to school, get a new certification, start applying for other jobs. Find a dream to pursue and go for it. It's a lot harder to take a risk with a job change when you have mouths to feed. But when you don't have kids, you have freedom to explore.

If work isn't where you want your legacy, consider building relationships with people you can have more time with now than you could if you had kids. Be someone's favorite aunt. Make cookies with your friends' kids. Get to know the widow who sits a few pews away from you in church. You might find an extremely satisfying friendship with a spunky old lady you'd hardly have known if you had to spend a bunch of time on play dates with other parents.

And you know what? There's an alternative to worrying about your legacy at all. There's a lot to be said for being someone who uses their life to appreciate the legacies others have already created or left. You could read a hundred books. Travel to every wonder of the world. Become a foodie. Visit every national park in the country. There are so many things the world has to offer. You could make it your goal to explore as much as you can.

It would be devastating to live your whole life and feel like you never added or appreciated anything really worthwhile in the world. Yet, it's not that hard to find ways to engage in and contribute to the world when you have time to do it.

Personally, I think it's kind of sad that a lot of parents believe their children are their only legacy. There are so many other ways to live a life with meaning and purpose, so many things you can do to make all your trips around the sun count. Put a little effort into figuring out what "legacy" means for you, and you might find that your legacy has been waiting for you all this time.

3. Learn how to self-soothe.

I recently read Lewis Carroll's *Through the Looking-Glass.* I'm so fascinated by the pool of tears Alice creates for herself at the beginning of the book. Mostly, I think Caroll's work is kind of trippy, but that pool of tears is a wonderful life analogy. It is easy to cry yourself a pool of misery deep enough it threatens to drown you. It's much harder to learn how to cry a pool of tears just big enough for you to float to the top of the pool and climb out.

Tip from a veteran: one of the best things you can let infertility do is teach you how to cry a pool of tears, then dry your own eyes and get out of the pool before your skin gets wrinkly. The ability to feel pain, self-soothe, and get on with living is so useful. Frankly, it's hard to learn a skill like that without experiencing pain, but you're going to have pain with infertility. You might as well get something out of it.

Initially, I wasn't very good at self-soothing. I was a wreck after that first miscarriage. Pain, however, is a great teacher. After we learned about our second miscarriage, I felt pretty numb. I was ten weeks pregnant, and I'd already seen the baby's heart beat. I couldn't believe she was now gone. I sort of stumbled out of the doctor's office not being able to see or feel anything. Then I let myself feel the sadness, and I cried. A lot. So did Malcolm. It was a rough night.

The next day, Malcolm took the day off. It was a beautiful, fall weather day. We spent it driving around, listening to our favorite playlist, talking about how pretty it was outside and also how sad we were. We said, "I love you" and "I hate this" and "I wanted that little girl" and "We'll get through this" and "I am so glad I'm going through this with you." We over-ate burgers, fries, and shakes at Five Guys. We played with our doggie at home and told her how much we love her, too.

The day after, I went to a surgery center for a D&C, appreciated the deep relaxation of anesthesia, and spent the afternoon sleeping on our living room couch. I remember all kinds of details from that day.

A few days later, I drove four hours away to meet a friend for a writer's retreat. We chatted a lot, but not about babies. We wrote a lot. I ate a lot of Cheez-Its and carbs, but I wasn't alone binge-eating on my couch.

The last morning of our retreat, we had coffee in a cafe, and two moms were playing with their babies there. That was also my thirty-eighth birthday and watching those moms made me sad again. I cried through a lot of the drive back to North Carolina. The tears felt cathartic. I knew something bad had just happened to me. I knew I was allowed to feel sad about that. I let myself feel sad when I needed to feel sad.

I already had a therapist. I was already on depression medications. I talked to my therapist about the miscarriage. I was thankful for that Wellbutrin.

I requested some space and privacy from our families for

the holidays. Malcolm and I got a real Christmas tree and had fun decorating it. We went low-key with gifts. I set boundaries I needed and avoided things I knew would hurt too much.

I bought a new goal-setting planner for 2020 and enthusiastically filled it out. In January, we started a new IVF cycle. In February, I published a new book.

I stored the sadness where it belonged and moved on.

Now, I remember the months after that miscarriage as a time when I lost something I desperately wanted but found a lot of light in the dark. The day immediately after the miscarriage was heartbreaking and also heartwarming. That is a vast difference from how I handled the first miscarriage, and it all comes down to my learning what works best for me when I need to self-soothe and cope with pain without either ignoring it or blowing it out of proportion.

Infertility comes with many lows, and you will probably feel anguish, grief, and disappointment. Those feelings won't go away on their own. There will be sorrow with every baby you lose, every embryo that doesn't implant, every negative pregnancy test. You will have to pass through those things, even when they cause you physical pain.

There's an art to feeling pain and not let it sink you. For me, doing so is about finding ways to put the pain next to things that remind me about how good life is. I lost a baby last year, and I hate that. It makes me feel so sad inside to think of that little angel I was supposed to get to cuddle and raise. But that season was still beautiful, those greasy burgers were still delicious, my dog was still pure wiggly butt joy, the anesthesiologist was still attractive, and I still have a supportive and loving husband who reaches for my hand in the car.

Beyond looking for the color in life when everything

feels gray, I also find that "getting back to normal" when I can is important for self-soothing. That doesn't mean switching off all the pain at once. I give myself grace these days when I need time to hurt. I've also learned there are things I can do that will make me feel like the world is still spinning when my heart wants to tell me it's not. There are cues to help my brain know I'm still surviving.

Malcolm and I both find that getting back to work is the easiest way to get back on track. It helps him to go back to the office and let his mind get lost in business that has nothing to do with infertility. It helps me to get back to my writing and get lost in a story that has nothing to do with infertility.

We are not entirely the same. I find that getting back to normal *social* events is much more difficult, especially with our families, because I cannot always cope with my own grief if I have to process the grief my family feels, too.

This is also part of self-soothing: knowing how you need to protect yourself while you heal. I need to protect myself from the sadness that other people feel for me, but the separation doesn't need to be permanent. I only need the time to wrap up my own grief well enough that I won't be bothered so much by someone else's pain.

So I allow myself to set the boundaries I need without guilt these days, too. This doesn't always make my family or Malcolm's happy. But I think this is one of those things you learn. Making someone else happy isn't your job when you get hit with another loss. That's their job. Your job is to give yourself what you need to heal.

That's my system. Feel the pain. Do things that are comforting. Remind yourself that life is beautiful. Get back to normal. Set boundaries where necessary. Give yourself grace when you need it.

That's how I've learned to manage grief and pain. The skills seem to apply not just to infertility lows but to any lows, too. I know this because I had to face more difficult lows in 2020 than I ever had before. (And more on that in Chapters Seventeen and Eighteen.) Again, though, infertility taught me how to stay strong in the face of loss. That's a major silver lining.

FINAL THOUGHTS ON STRENGTH TRAINING

Infertility can feel like a black hole in the middle of your life, sucking away everything you ever wanted. But you can choose to think of the empty space that remains as the place where you let other things in, and if you do that, you may find that your life can be richer than you ever believed.

We learn from overcoming difficult things. You can come away from infertility with a gain frame that helps you think positive in the darkest times, an ability to build a meaningful legacy that isn't dependent on children, and self-soothing and coping skills that will get you through far worse than this. You can look for the lessons infertility has to teach you, which may not be the same as the lessons it had to teach me.

Most importantly, you can choose to let your infertility define you as a sad, lonely, traumatized person, or you can choose to let it build you into a resilient, positive, interesting, strong person who can handle whatever life throws at them. I opt for Choice B. I hope you do, too.

CHAPTER SIXTEEN
Good People Say Bad Things

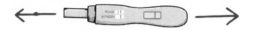

SANDY. IS. DONE.

It is April 2018, and I am just a little done. I'm a little fed up with infertility. I'm thirty-six. I've gone through all kinds of unsuccessful infertility treatments, and I am so tired of all the stupid things people say to people who are struggling with infertility. So, for National Infertility Awareness Week, I publish an article on Medium about what people should and should not say to someone going through infertility treatments.

It is incredibly cathartic, and I don't think I've ever regretted anything I said in that article. Much of what I wrote still holds true, and this is one issue I really haven't addressed yet in this book. Nevertheless, I bet that if you're struggling with infertility, you've heard people say all kinds of stupid things about it.

I bet some people have made you sad and others have made you spitting mad, and maybe sometimes you really want to hand those people a book and say, "Here, read this. Chapter Sixteen. Then never ever say that again, okay?"

So this is your resource. It's an updated and revised version of the article I posted on Medium in 2018, and it's for you and your well-meaning friends, family members, neighbors, co-workers, yoga buddies, and random grocery store acquaintances, all of whom probably think they have something useful to tell you about getting pregnant.

But first, some wisdom: if you struggle with infertility, people are going to say dumb things to you.

Even the smart people in your life will do it. They should know better, but they don't, and frankly, the whole "my infertility is none of your business" message isn't for everyone. It can feel alienating when people you care about know you're going through something really difficult but never feel like it's okay to say, "How are you doing?"

The truth, of course, is that infertility as a topic of conversation is a minefield. We all have different preferences for how much we are willing to talk. Our loved ones want to be there for us, but they often either say the wrong things or ignore the problem entirely because they are afraid they will say the wrong thing if they try to talk to us about it. And infertility is a very isolating problem, so never talking about it is bad for everyone and education is important.

The list below is a not-so-short list of things that, in my humble opinion, no one should ever say to someone who is going through infertility. It's based on my own personal experience, and everything you see here is something someone has said to me. My hope is to clear some of the mines from the field with this list, especially for anyone reading this book for the sake of a loved one. But before we get there, there are some things you, the person actually going through infertility, can do to deal with the issue of good people saying stupid things. Here's my advice:

INFERTILITY LESSON #17

1. Be explicit with your friends and family about how much you are willing to talk about your experience and make sure they know this is a work in progress. If you want to talk, tell them. If you want to keep quiet, tell them. You might change your mind about whether you want to talk later. Tell them that. If you aren't sure what you want right now, tell them that. Your loved ones aren't clairvoyant. If you want them to get it right, you have to tell them how.

2. Avoid assuming that people know what you want or that they are always going to get it right. They aren't. They want the best for you, and they aren't trying to hurt you when they make mistakes. So forgive your friends and family when they say something that hurts, even if they should know better. This could be a long road. You're going to need those people who care about you as you travel down it.

Basically, get used to gently and proactively guiding the people you care about around the land mines of infertility conversations. It will help you help them.

Now, for you loved ones …

HOW NOT TO TALK ABOUT INFERTILITY
Guidelines for Family & Friends

If you're reading this because you know someone going

through infertility treatments, and you want to avoid saying harmful things, then thank you. These guidelines are for you, and they are a list of things you need to think about when you talk about infertility.

As you go through the list below, you might find something that you've said. If that happens, don't feel terrible. Most of the things listed here have been said to me by smart, educated people who I respect, and always, more than one person has said these things. It's never just you.

Keep in mind that a list like this is highly personal. I think I'm naming things a lot of people going through infertility hate, but we are not all the same. What upsets me may not upset your neighbor who's going through infertility treatments. Pay attention and be a listener. You'll probably mess up sometimes, but if you're trying to look for cues about what you should and shouldn't say, you'll probably get it right more often than not.

Okay, here goes. These are the thirteen things you should never say to someone struggling with infertility. Starting with ...

1. "I can't even imagine what you're going through. My children are my whole life."

This is at the top of my list of the worst things to say to someone struggling with infertility because it is something many many many people are guilty of saying, and they have no idea it's wrong.

I don't mean to be nasty or unfeeling about this, but if your children are your whole life, you need to keep that secret to yourself. Definitely don't say something like that to someone struggling with infertility, but also consider dropping the statement entirely. Consider dropping the whole belief. Never say it to your own children. Tell them they bring you joy. Tell them you love them more than anything. But do not tell them they are your whole life. Because every time you say that, you send the message that children are the most important thing a person can possibly have, and if it turns out that your child cannot have children of their own, that's going to be a very difficult internal belief for your child to overcome.

When you go through infertility, your life perspective changes. You realize it is possible that you will not have children, and for a lot of people, that's a major loss. But if I am not able to have kids, should I tell myself that there is no way for me to live a whole, wonderful, joyful, fulfilling life?

Of course not. I need to believe that my entire life does not have to revolve around my children. That's the only way to get through this. I must think of myself as a complete person even if I never have kids, and it's bad for me to hear messages that tell me the opposite of that.

As a side note, if you truly do feel like your children are your whole world, you might want to get out and do some other things. Love your kids like crazy, but for their sake, do not make them the only interesting thing you have going on. It will be better for everyone if you have more depth to your life.

2. "Having children changes everything."

Not being able to have children changes everything, too. See (1) above. It can make you totally reevaluate your life purpose and change the way you expect to experience happiness. It can change your social circles and what rites of passage you are involved in. If you don't have children, you may not be invited to kid birthday parties. You probably won't ever face PTA politics. You'll never have empty nest syndrome. You may have to pay a stranger to take care of you as you age. You will not die with your children by your side. For a couple struggling with infertility, that's a lot to come to grips with.

Infertility changes everything.

But, you know ... life is full of things that transform us. Of course, having kids changes you, but that doesn't mean that a childless person has never had a transformational life event or that a childless person doesn't have wisdom of their own. You have your experiences, I have mine. I know things you don't know, and vice versa. There is no need for you to tell me that having children changed you, as if you're part of some club I can never get into. I'm part of a club you can't get into. So what? How about we focus on what we have in common instead of on what you think you have that I don't because you have kids.

3. "I tell my kids all the time that I want grand babies and I don't want them to wait to have them."

It is not your call if your kids have kids. Your kids don't owe you grandchildren, and it's never appropriate to pressure your children to have children of their own.

Even if you're only saying something like that because you just really don't want your kids to miss out on the joy that having kids brought you, you need to understand that you are potentially setting your own kids up for heartbreak when you say something like this.

You don't have to hide from your children that being a parent was meaningful for you, that you'd like them to have that experience, and that you'd love to have grand babies. However, as my wise ob/gyn once told me: no one gets to choose if they're going to have kids. So putting pressure on your kids to pull off a miracle because you really want it is terrible parenting on your part.

If you love your kids, leave room for the possibility that they won't want kids or won't be able to have them. If you fail to give them that space, and they later try to have kids and can't, how are you going to feel? Really incredibly shitty. That's how. Because you will have contributed to making something that's hard enough on its own even harder. Don't do this to your kids.

4. "Don't give up. I know someone who had a baby when she was 46."

Yep. I do, too. But even though there are people who are infertile for years and go on to have lots of kids naturally when they are older, there are also people who are infertile and never go on to have kids.

Let me repeat this very important truth: children simply aren't a guarantee. Just because someone else was able to have kids at a later age, does not mean I will be able to. You have no idea whether I can have children. You also do not know the burden I am carrying every time I try again. Who knows how that is affecting me? Maybe I don't have it in me to keep this up until I'm 46!

Also, I know that it is possible to have children at 46, but I struggled to have them at 36, so maybe it's petty, but I don't always want to hear about the person you know who got the miracle I want. It's not helpful.

5. "When are you trying again?"

Along the same lines as what I said in (4) above, infertility comes with costs you can't always see. Infertility treatments are hard on the body, the mind, and the wallet. It is not always financially possible for a couple to try another cycle of in vitro fertilization, especially if they are balancing the cost of one more try against the cost of something like adoption or a surrogate. Even if it is financially possible, the couple might have some other reason not to try a given treatment again, including emotional exhaustion.

It's difficult enough for someone with infertility to make the decision about when to stop. Don't be the person who adds pressure by asking when they're doing this again as if it's a foregone conclusion that they'll try until they have a baby or bust. It's not. It's also not your job to be part of this decision.

6. "You'll regret it if you give up."

Unlike (4) and (5), this line is usually said by someone who could have had children and regrets that they didn't, so it can be extra damaging because it carries a whiff of "wisdom." Note that this is not usually said by someone who tried to have children but ultimately couldn't. The difference is very very important.

In the first case, the person now wishes they had chosen the option of having kids, but they do not know what it's like to struggle to have them. They have never experienced getting to the point where you are physically, mentally, and financially incapable of doing more. They have no idea what someone who is going through infertility treatments is actually experiencing.

The person in the second case has experienced getting to the place where they do not have the ability to do anymore. They know it all too well, and they also know that everyone has a different tolerance for pain. I wish I could say I had unlimited resources, but I don't. There have been times when I simply couldn't do more. I don't know where my ultimate stopping point will be, but I can tell you that no matter where that point is, when you get to "enough is enough," that decision has not been made lightly.

Someone who has no sense of what going through

infertility treatments is like has no clue what someone who has will later regret. They should not be offering wisdom about it.

7. **"My cousin's neighbor's best friend's daughter's ballet teacher's grandma's accountant tried to get pregnant for years. Then she took beeswax mixed with crushed dried wasp wings and a dab of rubbing alcohol, and she got pregnant just like that! Have you thought of going to her witch doctor?"**

No, thanks.

Please never say this again.

But also, please try to remember that there are a million treatments out there, and the person you are talking to is probably already working with a doctor who is an expert in these treatments. The doctor is in the best position to guide your infertile family member or friend and help them find the best treatment for their body. And you're not their doctor, so for all you know, what you're suggesting could interfere with a treatment.

Furthermore, saying something like this is a lot like saying "you should keep trying, and here's how." It's bad enough to pressure someone into continuing to try infertility treatments when you don't know the cost burden of those treatments. It's practically self-righteous to put that pressure on and add a recommendation as to how the treatments need to be done. Good grief.

If you absolutely MUST bring something like this up, please do it like this: "I heard of an infertility cure. Would you ever want me to pass on information like that to you?" If the person you're talking to says "no," you should say, "okay," and let it go. But more often than not, you should just keep stuff like this to yourself. She doesn't need to know.

8. "Have you tried Clomid? That worked for me. And make sure that you talk to your doctor about adding estrogen patches. That saved my first pregnancy."

So in fairness, this isn't really a "you should never say it" kind of thing. But it's sort of a sibling to (8), and it can still be very hurtful because it can feel like someone telling you that she knows your body better than you do.

Fertility issues are difficult to diagnose, and there are a lot of reasons that someone might have trouble getting pregnant. Even if you have gone through this yourself and are on the other end, you don't know my body and, again, you aren't my doctor. What worked for you may not work for me. It is possible that I'll want to know about your experience, and if I do, I'll appreciate as much information as you can tell me. But also, I'll probably ask if I want your advice.

Best practice on this kind of thing? Offer your expertise with caution and ideally only if solicited.

9. "You just need to relax, and it will happen. Stop stressing!"

I cannot tell you how often I hear this, and sometimes I hear it from people who should know a lot better. I had an acupuncturist once who liked to say this to me. She was good at acupuncture and I was going to her because she advertised that acupuncture could cure infertility, so I tolerated it until I found myself practically in tears in her office one day because I was feeling that bad about how my stress was causing me not to be able to have babies.

I ultimately told her I would not be returning because of this. I hope maybe it sunk in for her that she was saying something horrible to me. Probably not. People tend to be oblivious about these things.

But of all the things people say that they shouldn't, this is the one that I've always found the most traumatic and difficult to forgive. It is so incredibly hurtful when someone says something like this because there is no way to interpret it except as victim blaming.

Now, is it right? Who knows? There are some links between stress and infertility,[59] but to tell someone that if they "just relax" they will get pregnant is terribly unhelpful. First, maybe you were able to "just relax" and get pregnant, but that might not work for me. Just because stress reduction helps some women doesn't mean that if I relax, my ovaries will start functioning exactly like they're supposed to.

Second, infertility can absolutely turn you into a stress ball, and being told that you're the person who is at fault for your infertility because you are too stressed definitely doesn't cause any *less* stress. When your body isn't doing what it's supposed to be doing, it's already hard not to feel guilt and shame over that. No one going through infertility needs to be made to feel worse about their body malfunctioning. To the extent stress contributes to infertility in any way, telling a woman to stop stressing is not likely to make her feel less stressed. So please, if you don't want to cause harm, don't go there.

10. "I understand what you're going through because I had it much worse."

Comparing who had it worse is almost always a bad idea when it comes to pain, no matter your intention. All you do when you tell another person that you understand because you had it worse is make the other person feel angry, misunderstood, and marginalized. Why would you tell them you had it worse if not because you want them to know their pain isn't that impressive? Why would you make their pain about you at all? This is not empathizing. This is bringing yourself into a space you were not invited to and then judging that space to be smaller than it actually is. It is not welcome.

I do not care how many miscarriages you had. I do not care how many IVF treatments you had. It does not matter if the person you are talking to has only had one miscarriage and you had ten. It does not matter if the person you are talking to has only gone through one IVF cycle and you've gone through twenty. It doesn't matter if your experience really was worse. It is never okay to tell someone that you understand what they are experiencing because you experienced the same thing times twenty.

We all experience pain in life, but it doesn't hit us exactly the same way or at exactly the same time. How do you know your experience was worse? Maybe you went through more IVF cycles than she did, but maybe she spent every penny she had on the one cycle she went through. Maybe you went through more miscarriages, but maybe she lost a child. Maybe on paper, it looks like you went through a million times worse, but maybe she's just not as resilient as you. Maybe the pain that hurt you hurts her worse. You have absolutely no idea how she's feeling because you're not living in her body and she may not be telling you everything anyway.

When someone tells you about something that is hurting them, don't make the mistake of trying to make them feel better by shifting the conversation to discuss your pain. The comparison will not help your loved one.

11. "Why don't you just adopt?" or "Why don't you just try a surrogate?"

There are a lot of ways that a person can acquire a baby. But with the exception of sex, almost all the ways you can get a baby are expensive, emotionally draining, barely covered by insurance, and not a guarantee.

Adoption can be competitive. It is also not for everyone. It's really great that there are wonderful parents out there adopting kids who need homes, but the person you are talking to may not have the financial resources to adopt or might simply not be ready to go there. It is not selfish to grieve the children that would have had your husband's beautiful eyes and your sharp wit. It is not easy to give up on the dream of having your own children, and not everyone is willing to adopt.

Surrogacy is complicated. There are a lot of legalities to consider. Even if you think it would have been nice to have your children without the pregnancy part, pregnancy is an experience that some women really want to have. It may be hard to give that up, too.

More importantly, there really is no "why don't you just" when it comes to infertility. There is no "one size fits all" solution. And there's much more out there than you likely realize if you're not knee deep in it yourself.

"Why don't you just try X?" is always a bad question. It's never "just" that easy.

I do get that people are also curious about these things, though. So consider this: if you are asking "why don't you just try X?" because you're making an assumption that "X" is easy, then don't ask the question.

If you're asking because you're curious and concerned—and the person you are talking to has made it clear that it is okay to talk to them about their infertility struggles—frame your question like this: "Do you think X could ever be an option?" That lets the other person know that you legitimately don't know much about "X" and opens up a much better discussion with far less possibility for pain.

12. "Have you seen that show on Netflix that is

vaguely related to reproduction? You'd love it."

There was a year in my life when I had multiple good friends tell me I needed to watch *Jane the Virgin* because I would love it. Good friends. People I dearly love and respect. Apparently the show's sense of humor matches mine in some way. But no, I have not watched *Jane the Virgin*, and I never will, because *Jane the Virgin* is about a woman whose doctor mistakenly artificially inseminates her during a checkup. I know that's supposed to be funny, but it's really not for someone going through infertility treatments.

Furthermore, the fact that the show is about a woman who gets pregnant means that watching it is likely to involve watching a show about pregnancy and babies. That's not something I'm dying to do. I also do not want to watch shows or read fiction about women going through infertility or miscarriages or anything related to reproduction. I'm experiencing it in real, non-fiction life. I don't need more of this for fun. Please don't suggest it.

13. "Do you know why you can't get pregnant?" or "Do you know why you miscarried?"

You know what? Even if I do, I might not want to talk about it. But more importantly, your job when you find out someone is struggling is not to be a problem-solver. Also, you could have the best of intentions when you ask something like that, and it is likely to come out as victim-blaming anyway. The person going through infertility doesn't hear you trying to help them figure out a way to get pregnant or not miscarry a second time. The person hears you saying "what did you do to cause your miscarriage?" and "what did you do to cause your infertility?" So don't say something like this. It's going to hurt the other person, not help them.

WHAT YOU CAN SAY

So what can you say to someone who's going through infertility treatments? Well, there is one thing. Here it is:

"I know you're going through something difficult. I want you to know I'm here for you, but I'm going to take your lead on this. We can talk if you want to talk, or we don't have to. All you need to do is tell me what you want."

If the other person has made it clear that they are willing to talk about their infertility, and you want bonus points, you could try something like this, too:

"How are you feeling?" or "How are things going?"

Open-ended questions are usually pretty safe, as long as you're listening for cues that the other person doesn't want to answer your questions today.

No matter what you do, you'll get it wrong sometimes, but on behalf of those of us struggling with infertility? We appreciate your attempts to get it right. Thank you for that.

PART VI
My Story Isn't Over

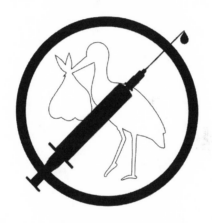

Honestly, I think God loves to give us more than we can handle. I think it's God's way of keeping things interesting and reminding us why our faith matters.

~ Me

CHAPTER SEVENTEEN
My Infertility Journey Almost Ends

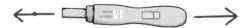

BEGINNING OF THE END

You know how at the end of a book series, the main character often takes a journey that forces her to revisit all the challenges that led her to the final battle? She has one last mountain to climb, but you get to see all the ways she's grown as she climbs it? She has to navigate a maze—again— but this time she knows where to find a map. She has to slay a dragon—again—but this time she has a magic sword.

That is sort of how my infertility journey went. I did everything, and then I had to do it all again a second time, and I've given you bits and pieces of my second run throughout this book. In this chapter, I'm going to give you the full account, start to finish, so you can see how I navigated infertility after I had some experience. This is my "infertility lessons in action" chapter, if you will.

There's a twist, though. As I write this final chapter, I'm almost eight months pregnant. I'm planning to release this book the week of Thanksgiving 2020 because I am so grateful for the baby I have on the way. I also set the week of Thanksgiving because we're expecting the baby to arrive on December 1, 2020, and I have no idea what my life will look like after that.

I guess I don't do anything the easy way, either. This has been, to say the least, a challenging pregnancy. More on that in Chapter Eighteen, though, when you learn why my story has an ambiguous ending. First, let's go back to how this pregnancy got started, and I'll walk you through what a good infertility story looks like.

THE START OF A NEW JOURNEY

It's late spring of 2018, and Malcolm and I still live in Georgia. We are out of embryos. Drugs and sex isn't working for us. If we want a baby, we only have two options left. Option one: we can start fresh with a new IVF cycle. That will mean egg retrieval and genetic testing and probably more diagnostic testing. We're not sure it will work. We're thirty-six now, and that's a significant difference in age from when we did our first egg retrieval at age thirty-three. Our track record is unimpressive. Why would we have success now with older eggs? Still, we're not sure we're ready to give up on IVF.

Option two is adoption, something we're even more nervous about. From the small amount of research we've done so far, we know that when people say, "But you can just adopt," they have no clue what they're talking about. We're savvier than we used to be. We don't know all the details, but we know adoption, whether we do it through the state or a private agency, will involve all kinds of classes and preparation, a comprehensive home study with a social worker who may actually look through our closets, and then an incredible amount of effort just to be put on a waiting list. After that, we'll pray that someone chooses us to be the parents of a baby plenty of other childless couples would be happy to parent, too.

So, do we choose difficult option one or difficult option two? Before we can decide, our lives get shaken up with our move from Georgia to North Carolina. It happens fast. Malcolm gets a job offer in May, and we're house hunting in North Carolina in June.

We ask our reproductive endocrinologist in Georgia if there is a doctor she would recommend to us in Raleigh. Turns out, she knows someone there. She emails the doctor while we're sitting in her office, which makes us feel good. We're getting a head-start on researching fertility clinics in Raleigh. We also have a friend who does research in reproductive endocrinology, and we ask if he has a recommendation for a doctor in Raleigh. Our friend names the same person our Georgia doctor recommended.

That's enough for us to feel like the universe wants us to try IVF one more time. We move into temporary housing in August 2018 in Raleigh, and because I know it can take some time to get hooked up with a new fertility clinic, I call the new clinic where the new doctor works while we are still living in temporary housing.

It's the week of August 20th, and the fertility clinic can't get us in for a consult with the doctor we want to see for two weeks. This is exactly why I called as soon as possible to make an appointment. We schedule the consultation for September 6, 2018.

Lesson learned: do not wait to get help.

In the meanwhile, I also make my first appointment with a psychiatrist in the area. I want a professional who can make sure I'm on a safe depression medication—or who can help me safely go off a depression medication—while I'm trying again to get pregnant.

We close on a new house in August, but I meet my new psychiatrist before then. I bet I'm one of his least dramatic patients. I have reliably taken one depression medication for years. I have no desire for either an increased or decreased dosage. I don't miss appointments, I usually show up on time, and what I want from this psychiatrist is just a professional who can help me if I need to make changes.

I'm probably boring as hell to him, but I feel like an all-A's student with this. I'm proactive about maintaining good mental health. I might be better at this than I am at flossing, and I'm the kind of person who gets neurotic about flossing. Gold star for me.

Lesson learned: before you start infertility treatments, find a psychiatrist to help you manage your depression meds while you're trying to get pregnant.

Malcolm and I meet our new reproductive endocrinologist in September, and we both like him right away. The doctor is personable, confident, and smart. He has reviewed the thick stack of medical records we asked our fertility clinic in Georgia to fax over. He doesn't seem to mind the high level of snark we bring to infertility appointments these days or our gallows humor, which is great, because that humor gets us through this.

Lesson learned: develop a sense of humor about this with your partner because you're going to need it.

Several other things happen in our initial meeting with

the doctor that make us feel good about this choice, too. Two things stick out for me.

First, the doctor notes that I have PCOS. I say something like, "Oh, do you think that's a sure thing? No one's ever formally diagnosed that for me." The doctor looks almost disappointed in the medical system, which I appreciate. I have always hated that no one ever wants to label what's going on with me. This doctor is willing to call it like he sees it. He says, "You have PCOS." Finally.

Second, the doctor recommends going straight to IVF and doing genetic testing on the embryos. However, he points out that it isn't clear why IVF hasn't worked for us in the past. It might not be the embryos.

"Sometimes, we don't know why someone isn't getting pregnant," he tells us. "It could just be bad luck." When we were starting infertility treatments, I might not have appreciated an honest statement like that. After all, this doctor is admitting that making babies isn't an exact science. Now, I know better. This realism is a sign that the doctor will never feed us any bullshit. He will do his best to help us, but he isn't a witch doctor miracle maker.

There's a factor for Malcolm, too. He suspects that the doctor is not too much older than we are (we are not young at this point) and that the doctor might be a car guy. We have no idea if any of this is true, but that's not the point. The point is that we both trust this doctor from the beginning, and that makes us feel good about working with him.

Lesson learned: find a reproductive endocrinologist you trust.

We schedule our first IVF "class" for October 2. At this clinic, the "class" is mandatory before starting an IVF cycle. During the class, a nurse sits down with just me and

Malcolm, explains how a fresh IVF cycle works at this clinic, tentatively schedules out appointments for our egg retrieval cycle, gives us a "protocol" for medications and injections, demonstrates how to do the injections, and asks us to sign various consent forms related to what we want done with all the embryos and eggs.

The class reminds us that we've done far too many of these cycles. The injection demo is boring. When the nurse takes us to the finance department to talk about money, we also feel that we've "been there, done that." Which is sad, because we are paying up front and out-of-pocket for this fresh IVF cycle, which our insurance does not cover. That's a $15,125 charge for the baseline and monitoring appointments, semen collection, egg retrieval, egg fertilization, biopsying up to five embryos for genetic testing, and later embryo transfer cycle.

The medications for the egg retrieval add up to $4,313, and we pay those costs to the specialty pharmacy that sends the drugs to us. The fertility clinic estimates that genetic testing will be about $2,000, and we will later pay that cost to the genetic testing company. We're going to rack up a lot of Chase Sapphire points, but we expected all of this.

Lesson learned: find out what your costs will be and figure out what you want done with any eggs and embryos that come from an IVF cycle before you start the cycle.

We walk out of that class feeling hopeful. There's something about starting fresh again (ha! Did you like that IVF pun?) with a new clinic and a new doctor in a new state. Who knows? This might even work for us. Maybe by winter of 2019, I'll be pregnant. Malcolm and I are excited about the possibility.

I'M STILL AN EGG FACTORY

My baseline appointment for the egg retrieval is sched-uled for October 22, two months after I first called the new clinic to get in for a consultation. There have been no delays on our part. We've scheduled everything as early as possible. Good fertility clinics are just busy places.

We are unsurprised by how long it takes to go from a first call to an actual infertility treatment cycle, and we have plenty of patience with this process. This is good timing for us anyway. Malcolm is busy with his new job, and I'm busy unpacking our stuff, getting to know Raleigh, and hooking up with other writers in the area.

Additionally, in the middle of October, I pinch a nerve and end up in debilitating back, shoulder, and neck pain for a few weeks. This zaps my energy, and I'm anxious not to be on any major pain medications during the egg retrieval, so I spend tons of time at a chiropractor's office that month.

Thankfully, my chiropractors are healing magicians, and my pain is at least tolerable by the time October 22 rolls around. I go in for that baseline appointment, start taking medications and injections, and proceed with many moni-toring appointments. I recall uncomfortable bloating and digestive issues from the first time I did an egg retrieval, so this time around, I'm incorporating more fiber than normal into my diet. Oatmeal every morning.

Lesson learned: eat lots of fiber during infertility cycles or face the wrath of bloating and constipation.

Before I know it, the day of the egg retrieval arrives. We're so good at waiting by now that I feel like hardly any time has passed. Malcolm takes the day of November 8, 2018, off and we go to the clinic for the procedure. I strip down, leave my clothing in a locker, put on a gown, and watch while a nurse inserts an IV for the anesthesia.

They walk me to the room where they do egg retrievals. It's a smallish room for a surgical procedure, but this feels a lot like the first time I did an egg retrieval. The nurses show me where to sit on the table, how far to scoot my rear toward the edge, and where to put my legs in the massive stirrups. This felt like such a loss of dignity forever ago. Today, I'm just thinking it's pleasant that this clinic has warm, thick blankets that they drape over me while I'm lying on the table. Truthfully, I'm quite comfy.

Lesson learned: dignity is about how you control your thoughts, not your body.

An attractive anesthesiologist (who I later remember vaguely as a middle-aged woman) puts oxygen tubes in my nose. I don't think they did that at the first egg retrieval, but they should have. Oxygen is blissful. Then the anesthesiologist says, "Think about something nice!" and the anesthesia hits my veins. I imagine hanging out in a castle set in one of my epic young adult novels, and as that tingling sensation spreads through me, my mind exits the room and enters a pleasant fantasy world.

I wake up half an hour later or so in a recovery area. This egg retrieval was a huge success. They retrieved 37 eggs. I do not have a problem with my egg supply. I munch graham crackers and drink apple juice while Malcolm tells me that the nurses said 37 was a very high number of eggs. We know from experience that the number of eggs you start with doesn't necessarily give you a million embryos, but it still feels like a win. They are going to fertilize all of the eggs.

I go home and sleep for the rest of the day, and the icky

part of the egg retrieval doesn't start for me until after that. Producing that many eggs takes a toll on your system. I don't need to do injections anymore, but I'm a little hyperstimulated. I need to stay super hydrated while my body bloats in reaction to the ovarian stimulation. I guzzle Gatorade all week while we wait to see what happens with the eggs that were retrieved.

Lesson learned: stock up on Gatorade before your egg retrieval and stay hydrated!

I get reports from the embryologist over the next few days. Of the 37 eggs retrieved, 28 were "mature" enough to be injected with sperm via ICSI.[60] Out of those 28 eggs, 25 fertilize, so we initially get 25 embryos from the egg retrieval.

That's a great number to start with, and we're cautiously optimistic. By the end of the week, only ten embryos are still standing. The other embryos have already arrested or are in that process, and they have to be discarded. Our initial IVF package only accounted for five embryos, but we want all ten frozen and biopsied for genetic testing. We pay the clinic an extra $500 to biopsy the extra five embryos, and the clinic sends samples from all ten embryos to a genetic testing company.

PREIMPLANTATION GENETIC TESTING

The genetics company is doing Preimplantation Genetic Testing (PGT) on our embryos, and, specifically, our embryos are being tested for chromosomal abnormalities, which is considered "Preimplantation Genetic Screening" (PGS) as opposed to "Preimplantation Genetic Diagnosis" (PGD). With PGS, they're screening for general chromosomal abnormalities. With PGD, they test for specific, known genetic mutations.[61] The cost ends up being $1,550, and it takes several weeks to get the results back.

Lesson learned: there's always more waiting.

It's not a problem for us. Malcolm is still getting settled at his new job, and I'm determined to self-publish my first book this year. We bury ourselves in work and don't obsess about those embryos.

I finally publish my book on November 27, 2018. It is a huge accomplishment for me. I've been working on that book since 2014. Which is not as long as I've been trying to have a baby, but still. It's a significant amount of time, and it took significant effort. Sometimes I think I learned that stamina from infertility. Writing a book takes a lot of patience, but less so than infertility treatments. In a way, infertility made me capable of publishing.

Probably more importantly, for now, writing is something I use to cope with the unpredictability of infertility. I have no control over what happens with that genetic testing. I have plenty of control over what happens to my book, which is a young teen epic fantasy sci-fi novel that I title, *Sassafras and the Queen.*

I hope the book does well. If it doesn't, I'll try again with another. This is yet another way I'm different because of infertility. I see failure as a valid option for my first book. But I don't see it as a permanent condition. If the book fails, I'll try again until I either succeed or decide to move on to some other venture with the wisdom I learned from my failures.

I'm incredibly proud of myself for publishing the book with this attitude. I could be sitting around, fretting over those genetic test results instead. Not gonna lie. I think this makes me a total infertility rockstar.

Lesson learned: infertility can make you a more capable, more resilient, less anxious person.

As it turns out, we get the genetic testing results back the same week I hit "publish." Four of the ten embryos are normal. The other six are not. I'm worried about this at first. Why are only 40% of our ten embryos normal? But I know enough to stay calm and do research. I'm now thirty-seven years old, and when I look up the statistics, I find that, on average, only 43% of embryos from women aged 35-37 are normal.[62]

Our doctor is not concerned by our results, either. At our next consultation, on December 20, he tells us there's no pattern with the abnormal embryos that would indicate any particular genetic problem that might explain why we've never had success with IVF before. Four is a lot of embryos to work with. We have a lot of chances for a pregnancy.

If this is a video game, I now feel like we've passed Level 1 (find a new clinic and become established with a new doctor) and Level 2 (egg retrieval and genetic testing). We can move on to Level 3, which we assume will be the embryo transfer itself.

THE "ABNORMAL ABNORMALITY"

A person's body can change a lot in a year, and before we start our IVF cycle in the new year, our doctor wants to do a saline ultrasound just to make sure my uterus looks good. Then we can start a frozen IVF cycle and transfer one of our good, genetically normal embryos to my uterus.

Unfortunately, the doctor also wants to repeat the Endometrial Receptivity Analysis (ERA). That was one of the two worst diagnostic procedures I had to do before. It will require us to do a fake embryo cycle. That means I have to go through all the estrogen, the progesterone shots, and the monitoring appointments without any chance at pregnancy. Instead of actually completing an embryo transfer, the doctor will then perform a uterine biopsy that will hurt like hell, and he'll send the sample to a lab for analysis.

I am not dying to do this again, but the first ERA results weren't as conclusive as the doctor would have liked, and he feels that it would be worth repeating. So even though it sucks to have to do this again, I agree.

The test is too short for anesthesia, so I ask for a Xanax prescription to get through the test. The doctor has no problem with my request, but the nurse writes me a prescription for Valium instead, which is significantly more relaxation than I need to get through one painful snip. It's okay. I know how to advocate for myself. I just hand the prescription back and tell her I need Xanax, not Valium, and they rewrite it.

Lesson learned: advocate for yourself when you need to.

I fill the prescription, but on the day of the procedure, I don't take it. I do not recommend not taking perfectly good drugs that will help you in a situation like this, and I blame my husband for making me feel like I shouldn't be taking any drugs I "might" not need. That's his weird anxiety, not mine. I should have taken the Xanax.

Still, I get up on that examination table without the Xanax and try to relax as the doctor threads various tools through my cervix so that he can snip out part of my uterus. It's painful—as painful as I remember from the first time—for a few seconds, and then it's over. But I don't cry or freak out. I only cramp up and bleed a bit later. The doctor says I did well.

"A lot of women cuss," he tells me.

No kidding. But I walk out of the office that day feeling like I've triumphed over fertility diagnostic tests. I have conquered the waiting game. I have conquered the pain game. I'm a freaking warrior.

Lesson learned: to manage pain or have patience, you must know how to relax when you can't control your environment.

While the ERA goes well, the saline ultrasound reveals scar tissue, probably from the D&C I had years ago. The doctor says he can remove that tissue with a hysteroscopy. He says this like it's no big deal. A hysteroscopy is the other of the two worst diagnostic procedures I've experienced. That was the procedure that involved the incredibly long needle, the medical equipment that stalled, and the cold sweat. But I learn that this clinic assumes a patient will need anesthesia for a hysteroscopy.

Oh. Thank. God.

The hysteroscopy takes place at a surgical center, and another hot anesthesiologist (I think this one might be a blond man) gives me the good drugs. Because of this, I am unaware that the hysteroscopy takes longer than expected. But I wake up in a recovery area with a full bladder and some pain. The doctor is there, as is my husband, and the doctor explains that while he was able to cut out some scar tissue, he also had to insert a catheter and fill my bladder with saline to see my uterus better. As it turns out, my uterus has some "abnormal abnormalities."

That's bad.

I'm too groggy to discuss it in more detail right then, but

Malcolm and I go home feeling pretty lousy about the whole thing. Does this mean we won't be able to do the IVF after all? The doctor calls us the next day and tells us that what he saw makes him think I may have adenomyosis. Adenomyosis is like endometriosis but trickier to diagnose. It's what happens when your endometrial lining starts growing into the muscle tissue of your uterus, and because it happens in the muscle tissue, it's hard to see.[63]

As the doctor talks, I realize that I may have had this condition for years. After my first hysteroscopy in 2015, I was told my uterus was "heart-shaped." I didn't think anything of that at the time. It wasn't supposed to be a problem. But was that the adenomyosis? I've also had some issues with painful sex, especially in deeper positions. I don't talk about this because painful sex isn't exactly casual conversation material. However, it turns out that adenomyosis can cause painful sex because it causes your uterus to become enlarged. The doctor sends me for an MRI to confirm the adenomyosis.

Lesson learned: there's always another test and there's always something new to learn.

When we next talk to the doctor, he confirms the adenomyosis diagnosis and tells us that adenomyosis does not always affect a woman's ability to get pregnant. Still, since we've had a "long road," he thinks we should try a treatment that could reduce the effects of the adenomyosis. The treatment is three months of Lupron Depot shots, which, he explains, will put my body into an immediate—though temporary—menopause, cutting off my estrogen supply. Since endometrial tissue grows on estrogen, this will hopefully shrink my uterus back down and make it a better environment for an embryo.

It's an option we don't want to consider, for two reasons.

The first is timing. If I start the Lupron Depot in February, the earliest we can start our IVF cycle is May. That's three extra months of waiting, and we *are* good at waiting, but we've been working with this clinic now since August 2018 and it's already January 2019. Haven't we waited enough?

To complicate matters, we've been planning a road trip for May 2019. It's not just a little trip we can reschedule. It's a huge car rallye involving a large group of people. We've already put a non-refundable deposit down on that trip, and we're really looking forward to it. When we first signed up, we never dreamed that it would conflict with an IVF cycle, but now it does. We can't start a frozen transfer cycle during that trip. So if we do the Lupron Depot shots, we will have to delay them another month and wait to start the cycle in June. That's four months longer than we wanted to wait to start the frozen transfer cycle.

The second reason we're reluctant is that Lupron is a heavy-duty drug, and the side effects could be unpleasant. I'll have hot flashes, vaginal dryness, and potential memory loss. That last one scares me the most, but the doctor assures me that these side effects will be temporary. I'll have a few potentially unpleasant months, but then, hopefully, my uterus will be in perfect condition for our best embryo.

Malcolm and I discuss this, and ultimately, we decide that we've experienced too much failure not to pay attention to the doctor's recommendations despite our reluctance. I'll do the Lupron Depot shots, and we'll do our frozen transfer cycle in the summer. In the meanwhile, we'll distract ourselves with that road trip. At least I won't be pregnant while we're zipping around Utah in a tin can with no airbags. Silver linings, right?

There's another silver lining, too. Once I'm on the

Lupron Depot shots, I discover that my body is totally fine with menopausal side effects. The hot flashes seem minimal to me. I don't notice vaginal dryness. I'm a little forgetful for the first month, but then my brain seems to adjust. I get significantly fewer migraines, and I feel more energetic. Maybe my body hates estrogen. I decide the experiment was a good one, and I'm glad we did it.

Lesson learned: acquire a gain frame about your infertility.

SHATTERED DREAMS

We get to June, and now we can finally schedule that frozen transfer cycle. I order meds and go to my baseline appointment for the frozen cycle on June 17, 2020. The embryo transfer will be July 12, and we are extremely optimistic. We have done everything right. Everything. All those tests and all that prep and all that waiting must surely have paid off. This was our best embryo, my post-Lupron Depot uterus, and a perfectly timed IVF cycle. Plus, we've done so many many cycles before. Surely luck will be on our side this time?

On July 22, I go in for the pregnancy test.

It is negative.

We are crushed.

Lesson learned: the odds are still against you.

It's a shitty time for a negative pregnancy test. My entire family is getting together in Michigan next weekend for my grandmother's 90th birthday. *All* of my cousins have kids. All of them. There will be kids swarming the place.

Additionally, I'm not sure my parents will ever get over

that they don't have grandchildren of their own yet, but one of my cousins has a little girl who lives close enough that they can dote on her like she's a substitute grandchild.

Most of the time, that little girl is a huge blessing for me. The weekend of the birthday party, not so much. It's always hard to be around adorable little kids after a negative pregnancy test. It's extra hard to watch your mom give attention to someone else's incredibly sweet toddler a week after a negative pregnancy test.

I struggle to smile at that party, and I don't think anyone knows what to say to me. I have the sense that they all see me as a walking tragedy. I try to forgive the things people do say when it stings. They're all doing the best they can. My infertility woes aren't their fault.

Lesson learned: forgive your family for having no clue how to deal with your infertility and love them anyway. They love you.

I console myself with the thought that at least the pregnancy didn't end in a miscarriage. That would have been so much worse. But I've already had my miscarriage. I don't anticipate having another.

Malcolm and I start a new frozen IVF cycle with the next embryo as soon as we can. Our baseline appointment for that cycle is August 19, 2019. Our embryo transfer is September 13. The doctor adds estrogen patches to my protocol this time, and I add acupuncture treatments, and I swing back and forth between hope and hurt as the cycle begins. I write a novella in August and another in September to stay calm.

September 23 is the day of the pregnancy test, but I don't feel pregnant at all. I go in for the test, let them draw my blood, head to a Panera Bread for a smoothie, and brace for a negative.

The doctor calls me before I've left the Panera.

The test is positive.

I am so stunned, I almost don't believe him. I'm pregnant. And there's no questioning it this time. My HCG numbers are nice and high. This is amazing. This is incredible.

Malcolm and I are both thrilled. We spend the next several weeks looking at baby furniture and talking about names. It's a little girl. I want sweet girly furniture. Malcolm wants to hang one of those crystal chandeliers in her room. We can't get over that this is finally happening.

Then disaster strikes. I fly out to California to co-facilitate a two-day negotiation training with a colleague for the training company I used to work for. I assure Malcolm that flying doesn't cause miscarriages. It doesn't. I'm spotting a little tiny bit, but I call the fertility clinic, and they tell me not to worry unless I'm soaking a pad in an hour. Since I'm not, there's no reason to think I'm putting my baby at risk by flying to California for a short gig. I'm confident that this is fine.

I have a good time at the training. I haven't done this in a while, but I still enjoy negotiation training, and it's nice to see my colleague again. Then at the end of the second day of the training, I'm standing in the front of the room, making my concluding remarks, when I feel that something is leaking from my body.

I confuse my colleague by rushing immediately to the ladies room after the training ends and without saying goodbye to our client contacts. But I am gushing blood, and I'm sure I'm miscarrying the baby. That's what the Internet tells me. Bleeding during your first trimester equals miscarriage.

It is all I can do to get through the next couple of hours

without completely freaking out. I'm at a work event. I can't fall apart. I'm already checked out of my hotel room, so I have to find my suitcase and change my underwear in the ladies room, which, thankfully, is empty now that our training is finished.

I tell my colleague what's happening, call Malcolm, and call my fertility clinic. But I'm in California, and it's now six o'clock. My fertility clinic in Raleigh is closed. I try the emergency line but can't get in touch with anyone. Should I go to the hospital? The bleeding is steady—definitely a miscarriage—but it doesn't seem to be horror movie blood. I have no idea what to do. I'm supposed to be taking a red-eye flight home that night. I want to go home. But am I at risk of hemorrhaging out?

Thankfully, my colleague knows an ob/gyn, and we're able to get that person on the phone. The doctor kindly tells me that I'm in for a rough night but that no, I probably won't hemorrhage out on the plane.

My colleague, who is a saint, drives me to a pharmacy, where I pick up heavy-duty pads. Then I change out of my business clothing and into yoga pants at her house before she takes me to the airport. I take the flight back to Raleigh, and in the morning, I go straight from the airport to the fertility clinic, where my husband meets me.

You don't need an appointment when you're bleeding like I am, and the clinic gets me in right away to see the doctor for an ultrasound.

I'm not miscarrying. The baby is still there. She even has a fetal heartbeat now. Guess what? Google doesn't know everything. What I have is a subchorionic hematoma, which is bleeding that occurs between the uterus and the placenta or outer fetal membrane.[64] This happens sometimes, but it is not necessarily linked to miscarriage. It just looks scary.

Lesson learned: don't go to Google for advice about your reproductive system.

My doctor puts me on pelvic rest (no lifting, no sex, no exercise beyond light walking) and says this should resolve itself. I go in for two more appointments at the fertility clinic that October. Both times, the baby is fine, and although I do bleed a little more over those weeks, the hematoma does seem to resolve.

Finally, I graduate out of the fertility clinic. Malcolm and I make an appointment to see an ob/gyn for the first time on November 6, 2019. This is week ten of my pregnancy, and we've never gotten this far.

I'm so incredibly excited about this "graduation." I don't feel well the day of the appointment, though—I have a migraine headache the whole time—and it's a long, tiring appointment. We wait to be called back so the nurse can take my vitals. We're moved to another waiting room, where we wait to be moved to the doctor's office, where we wait for the doctor himself for a long time.

Once we're finally talking to the doctor, there's a lot of history to go over. We talk for at least thirty minutes. But then, we're through all the boring, introductory stuff, and we get to the part where a nurse takes us to an exam room so we can see the baby on the ultrasound machine.

I take off my jeans and sit on a table under a sheet, and Malcolm and I wait another fifteen minutes for the doctor to return so he can do an ultrasound and we can see the baby again. Those fifteen minutes feel like forever.

At last, the doctor comes into the room with the nurse. This is a transvaginal pelvic ultrasound since it's still so early in the pregnancy. I lean back and watch the monitor while the doctor inserts the ultrasound wand.

There's quiet for a while.

I don't really understand what's happening. I can see what looks like a baby on the monitor. That little peanut. That's our baby girl. So what's happening that the doctor doesn't seem happy? Why is he so grim as he moves the wand around? What is he looking for?

Then he says, "I'm sorry, there's no heartbeat."

The baby has died.

Lesson learned: miscarriage pain is awful.

THE BEST WORST DAY

I'm in a daze as we leave the doctor's office. It's a Wednesday evening. Malcolm and I both cry a lot that night. The doctor can't do the D&C until Friday, but Malcolm takes off Thursday because he doesn't want me to be alone.

It's beautiful outside that Thursday, and we have a beautiful day together, despite the tragedy. We take care of each other. We don't work much. We are grateful for what we have, even in the midst of this loss. Because of this, we both remember that Thursday later as one of our best days. We're in the middle of a tragedy, but at least we're together.

Lesson learned: take comfort in your partner when infertility hurts the most.

I am supposed to be driving back to Georgia this weekend for a family gathering at my aunt's house. My parents and my brother will both be there, and they all arrive on Friday. The four of us rented an AirBnB, and we were all going to be staying together for the weekend. I would have been eleven weeks pregnant this weekend and almost to the end of a first trimester. I was planning to tell my family about the baby at the gathering. I was so excited to surprise them. Monday morning, I was supposed to be heading up into the mountains for a writer's retreat with a friend. It was going to be a whole thing.

I can't do the whole thing now. I'm not going to be able to drive Friday. You can't drive the day of a D&C. That's a surgical procedure that involves anesthesia, and it's not safe to drive on a day you've been put under. Also, Malcolm wasn't coming with me for any of this, so now I have no idea what to do. Do I tell my family? Do I try to make it to Georgia on Saturday? I stall and tell my family I have a migraine headache Friday and can't make it but that I might be able to drive down Saturday.

I'm calm the morning of the D&C, and it goes well. No complications. The doctor says, "This wasn't your fault. There was nothing you could have done to prevent this." Malcolm drives me home. I sleep for the rest of the afternoon. We are still very sad, but I am not ashamed.

Lesson learned: a miscarriage is not your fault.

Friday night, I still don't know what to do about my weekend plans. Malcolm tells me to get a plane ticket for Saturday morning. I do, except then I can't go through with it. He's crushed, too, and I don't want to abandon him the day after the D&C. I cancel the plane ticket, and early Saturday morning I call and tell my parents the truth. I tell them I just miscarried a little girl. They cry. I have to tell the rest of my family the same. It's horrible. I shouldn't have bothered trying to protect them. They were going to find out one way or another.

By Sunday, Malcolm and I are both feeling a little better, or at least we know we need to start getting back to any normalcy we can find. I finally make the drive to Georgia so that I can see my family for a day. It's a short visit, but I think it's best this way. It's hard for my family to know what to talk about, and they are all so disappointed for me. I try to stay positive, but I'm devastated, and being with my family is a reminder of what happened. I'm glad this won't be a long visit.

Monday morning, I drive into the mountains for that writer's retreat. This is very good for me. The friend meeting me there knows about the miscarriage, but she doesn't have kids, and she's the type of friend who can manage to avoid treating me like I'm a tragedy, even in the middle of something like this. Plus, we do a good job motivating each other to write. I get a lot of work done on a book I'm drafting, and we have plenty of things to chat about that are related to our publishing endeavors, not my miscarriage. It's two and a half days of relief from my grief, and I think that allows my brain some rest.

Lesson learned: keep your old friends, but make friends with new people who don't have kids, too.

The miscarriage doesn't really hit me again until Wednesday. That's the morning my friend and I have coffee at that local cafe and end up sitting near two women who are talking about babies and cuddling one right in front of us. During the six-hour drive back up through the mountains to Raleigh, I alternate between enjoying the beauty of a fall drive, singing along to the radio, and sobbing. I let myself do all of that. I have a lot of grief to process. I don't see any need to rush it.

But I have better coping mechanisms generally these days. I don't beat myself up for crying or having grief. I don't tell myself I caused any of this. I didn't. Something atrocious happened to me, but it wasn't my fault. It's okay for me to feel bad. It's okay for me to need some time and space to recover.

I'm *nice* to myself for the rest of November and December. I set some boundaries. I tell my family that I need a break from the holidays this year. I love my family, but the thought of opening presents on Christmas morning or trying to look happy while shoveling down stuffing feels like too much.

Malcolm still wants to see his family, so his parents do come down for a week after Christmas. This is not something I have the energy for, and I spend a lot of that week in my office, working on my books. I don't mean to be rude, but I decide it's not my job to worry about how this makes them feel. My job right now is to recover. That's it.

Lesson learned: grieve how you need to grieve, soothe how you need to soothe, set boundaries how you need to set them.

Thankfully, I had enough foresight before we started IVF treatments in the summer to find a good therapist. So I don't need to find anyone new for support as the holiday season hits us. And I'm still on my Wellbutrin, which is a huge help.

Lesson learned: find a therapist before you start IVF treatments.

A NEW YEAR

January 2020 arrives. We have two more embryos left, and Malcolm and I plan to do both those IVF cycles this year. I feel very much that completing these last IVF cycles is something we are only doing because we need to give those little souls their chances at life. But my expectations are low, and I have a different kind of hope this year. I figure that even if I miscarry both embryos, this will at least all be over by January 2021. Either I'll be pregnant by then, or I'll have a newborn, or we'll be moving on to adoption. There is an end in sight.

I start thinking about this memoir. It's time for this infertility journey to conclude. We can start a new journey when this is over. Adoption is something I'm a little afraid of, but I'm so much stronger and more resilient than I was before all this began. I can handle whatever comes next.

I think I know what's coming next.

Ha.

You never know what's coming next.

CHAPTER EIGHTEEN
The Ambiguous Ending

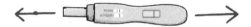

IT SHOULD HAVE ENDED THERE

My memoir should have ended there at the end of Chapter 17. Or at least I thought it should. When I first started thinking about this memoir, I was anticipating an ending that read something like this:

February 2020, one of our two remaining embryos fails. April 2020, we do our final IVF cycle with our last remaining embryo. We get pregnant, then miscarry. It's devastating, but we get through it. We head to Napa Valley to drink red wine and decompress after nearly a decade of infertility. We regroup in the fall and start the adoption process.

But 2020 was the year of the apocalypse, and nothing went the way I expected it to go. Nothing went the way anyone expected it to go. I didn't expect to be pregnant at the end of this story. I definitely didn't think the ending of this memoir would still be "ambiguous." It is, though, and so, my infertility journey is not quite over thanks to 2020.

Here's what happened to us this year.

I KNOW HOW THIS GOES

It is January 2020. After my miscarriage in the fall, the doctor recommended that I not start another IVF cycle until my body had gone through at least one normal cycle first. After a D&C, your body bleeds for a little while, then stops, and your cycle is supposed to start up again. I went through that in November, and my next cycle still hasn't started. The doctor told me to call the clinic if I hadn't had a period by the new year (remember, fertility clinics slow down around the holidays). On January 2, 2020, I call the clinic to tell them my period hasn't started. I anticipate that they'll want me to take birth control for a few weeks, maybe do a few more tests, then start the next cycle in February.

Sure enough, the clinic gives me a birth control prescription to take for a couple of weeks. They also schedule a saline ultrasound for January 29 and my FET "class" (the appointment where a nurse will plan out my next cycle with me) for February 3, 2020.

I was totally right about the timing. I pat myself on the back for being so smart about all of this.

Unfortunately, the saline ultrasound shows that there's scar tissue in my uterus. Well, what else is new? I'm going to need yet another hysteroscopy before I can begin IVF again. I'm told that I can start the IVF cycle a week after the hysteroscopy, but there are always reasons for delays. In this case, the doctor's next availability for the hysteroscopy is a few weeks into February, and my husband is traveling a lot this month for work and can't make the doctor's first available date for the procedure. We are unable to schedule the hysteroscopy until February 18. That's a few weeks later than I'd hoped to start the cycle, but it's okay. It's only a few weeks.

Thankfully, the hysteroscopy goes well. The doctor removes some scar tissue, and my uterus looks good enough that he tells my husband this before I'm awake from the surgery. He's gone by the time I'm up in recovery. I see this as a great result. There were no "abnormal abnormalities," so we had nothing interesting to discuss.

I go to the clinic for my baseline appointment on February 26. It has been two months since my call to the clinic on January 2, but I'm zen about it. So far, things are going exactly as unpredictably as planned.

I repeat my 2020 mantra to my husband while we start the cycle. "This will all be over by 2021. This cycle will work or it won't. But even if we miscarry, we'll be able to move on to our last cycle before the end of the year. We'll know how this ends by December 2020."

A GLOBAL PANDEMIC

We're old pros at IVF cycles. This is, after all, our 7th embryo transfer. If you count the two mock cycles we did, it's our 9th time doing progesterone shots. We are so experienced that I can do the shots myself if I need to.

I need to. Malcolm has to be gone for work a few days at the beginning of our IVF cycle. I am trying to stay stress-free during this cycle, so no travel for me. I've also banned visits from any parents until the cycle is over, and I'm doing acupuncture at least once a week, attending "gentle yoga" classes, and trying to eat decently healthy.

I'm expecting a negative pregnancy test result anyway. Honestly, I'm even kind of hoping for one. That would be much easier than another miscarriage. But I'm still trying to keep up a positive attitude. I keep busy, too. I publish another book in February. I have several more planned for 2020 alone. I have great expectations for the year in terms of my writing.

But there *is* this one thing that I didn't count on. The coronavirus. Initially, I don't take Covid-19 very seriously. Malcolm talks about how he thinks it's going to be a big deal, but that's casual dinner conversation for us through most of February. I dismiss sensationalist stories we read that tell us to stock up on toilet paper and frozen meat. A major pandemic sounds far-fetched to me. Malcolm and I both make Costco runs in late February anyway, and we independently buy extra toilet paper, but that's just in case. Mostly, we're focused on the IVF cycle.

As we all learn, though, Covid-19 is a real threat. By the week of March 9, 2020, we're nervous about it affecting our IVF cycle. Our embryo transfer is scheduled for March 20. We're less than two weeks away from that date, but Covid-19 keeps spreading. What if I get pregnant and then get covid? Will that hurt the baby? What if I get pregnant, and we need to keep doing progesterone shots but suddenly drugs aren't available like they used to be?

We email our doctor to ask him what he thinks. Should we cancel this cycle? We don't want to. We certainly don't want any more delays. But would it be safe to move forward?

The doctor thinks drugs like progesterone and estrogen are unlikely to become unavailable because they aren't hard to make. He says that we don't know exactly what covid does to pregnant women, but the illness seems to be respiratory, which shouldn't cause massive harm to a baby. He thinks we can move forward. We decide to move forward.

On March 11, 2020, the World Health Organization declares Covid-19 a global pandemic.[65] On March 13, the president of the United States declares a national emergency.[66] We are *one week* away from our transfer date. We bite our nails and worry.

On March 17, only four days before our transfer, the American Society for Reproductive Medicine (ASRM) issues a set of guidelines for fertility clinics recommending the following: "Suspend initiation of new treatment cycles, including ovulation induction, intrauterine inseminations (IUIs), in vitro fertilization (IVF) including retrievals and frozen embryo transfers, as well as non-urgent gamete cryopreservation" and "Strongly consider cancellation of all embryo transfers whether fresh or frozen."[67]

On March 18, we get a call from the receptionist at our fertility clinic, informing us about the ASRM recommendation and asking if we would like to cancel our cycle. It isn't required, but given the recommendations, they're offering cancellation to everyone.

I ask questions like, "When would we be able to start again?" and "Will any of our money be refunded?" The receptionist has no answer to either of these questions. We ask to speak to the doctor, who does his best to help us without really knowing how to answer our questions either. We don't know exactly how long this crisis might last. We don't know how bad it's going to be. We don't know what will happen if I get Covid-19. We don't know much of anything. No one does.

All the doctor can tell us for sure is that the clinic won't shut down. They'll always be open to serve existing patients.

This decision is up to us, and we have to make it based on a serious lack of information.

Malcolm and I talk it over. We're *three days* away, and this is one of the last cycles we expected to go through, ever. If we cancel the cycle, we have no idea when we might be able to start again. It could take a whole year. That's a major delay, even for people like us who are used to delays. By then, I'll be 39. That's not going to make getting pregnant easier.

We decide to move forward.

We get a call the day before the transfer from the embryologist. This is a standard call. They confirm that we want to unfreeze one embryo. We say yes.

The day of the transfer, we show up at the clinic, and the clinic turns Malcolm away. New policy. Only the patient is allowed into the back for the procedure.

This is a big big deal for us. IVF creates a huge separation between your partner and the actual potential pregnancy. Being there in the room while the embryo is transferred is emotionally significant for Malcolm. If the cycle fails, that will be the *only time* he ever gets to see the embryo alive in any way.

Why didn't they tell us about this policy yesterday? If we had known, we might have canceled the cycle. At the very least, if they'd given us any notice, we might have come up with an alternative, virtual way for Malcolm to be there. Now, my bladder is super full, I've just had my pre-transfer acupuncture appointment, and the embryo is unfrozen. If we don't go forward at this point, we'll lose the embryo, and these are long before the days of Zoom virtual meeting domination. We have no easy way to video conference Malcolm in for the procedure.

We have to go forward.

I'm a little angry. Malcolm is very angry. We understand that covid is life or death for some people, but this IVF cycle is life or death for our embryo. How could they change a policy like this between the time when they unfroze the embryo and the time we showed up at the clinic less than twenty-four hours later? Obviously, the whole world is facing a crisis, and everyone's figuring things out, but this is unacceptable.

Yet, I beg Malcolm not to create the kind of scene I know he wants to. If he does, I'm afraid we'll be kicked out, and that would be even worse than what's happening now. He goes and sits in his car while I do the transfer alone. It's extremely upsetting. I'm sure that this stress will prevent the cycle from working, if we ever had a chance to begin with, and I try to keep calm, but it's just not possible to fix this.

I have an acupuncture appointment right after the transfer. Thankfully, it's in the same building as the fertility clinic. I return to the parking lot to say goodbye to Malcolm first and see how he is. He is not okay. He is enraged. This makes me feel even more stressed. I go back inside for acupuncture feeling like I somehow caused the clinic to turn my husband away when really, this is a massive global problem showing up in our backyard. At least they allowed us to do the transfer. We discover later that some clinics just shut their doors.

Acupuncture does not make me feel any more relaxed. I've worked with the same acupuncturist for weeks now, but today, schools in Raleigh are all shut down. My normal acupuncturist has children, so she wasn't able to come in, and the person I have instead doesn't do things quite the same as the acupuncturist I'm used to. In particular, this acupuncturist must have a very different sense of internal body temperature than I have. The room is far too cold.

I lay on the acupuncture table, freezing and stressed and

trying not to cry. My infertility journey has prepared me for a lot, but a national emergency, a global pandemic, and my fertility clinic turning my husband away at the door are all factors I've never dealt with before.

I cannot imagine this cycle will end in a pregnancy.

BUT WAIT. IS THIS SUCCESS?

For the next ten days, we wait for our pregnancy test and the world falls apart. Malcolm's office closes, and he begins working from home. He makes jokes with colleagues about trading toilet paper for firewood, and I get upset because toilet paper is *not* something I want to be without if I happen to get pregnant.

I go to one more acupuncture session, but I'm otherwise in for the duration. No more in-person coffee shop writing. No more grocery store runs. I'm afraid even to walk around the park with a friend. Malcolm and I watch the news like everyone else and wonder if things will ever be the same again.

In the meanwhile, I don't feel any different, and I'm still expecting this to be a failed cycle. Usually, when I do IVF cycles, I wait until the pregnancy test the clinic does, and I don't "cheat" with at-home pregnancy tests. After all, the sticks you pee on can be inaccurate, and I don't want to assume I might be pregnant based on those tests.

This time, what I am most afraid of is being hopeful the day of the pregnancy test if there's no chance whatsoever. So I have a whole pack of cheap pregnancy test dipsticks, and I start using them two days after the IVF transfer. I am expecting them to show me one line every day until the day of the pregnancy test, when we can confirm that the test was negative.

There is only one line on Sunday. Same on Monday and Tuesday. On Wednesday, I think I see something where a second line would be on the pregnancy test, but it's like seeing a ghost. I try not to think much of it. Same thing Thursday, except on Thursday, Malcolm thinks maybe he sees something, too. It probably doesn't mean anything.

Friday there's a faint second line. Saturday, there's a stronger second line. Sunday, there's a very visible second line. Our pregnancy test is Monday, March 30, 2020.

The test is positive.

I'm pregnant. In a pandemic.

But it's about to get worse.

THREATENED MISCARRIAGE

Now that I'm pregnant for a third time, I'm always waiting for another miscarriage to occur. I start spotting a week after the pregnancy test, and I suspect a subchorionic hematoma. This is what my doctors think caused my miscarriage in the fall, and I'm sure it means this pregnancy is doomed, too.

There's no solid research that says you can make a subchorionic hematoma worse by exercising, walking, lifting, or anything else. However, I have recently learned that my mother bled while she was pregnant, and her doctors told her to keep her feet up during the day. She had two babies, so I feel maybe I should pay attention to this wisdom, even if it isn't backed by science. I rest as much as I can, avoid long walks, and keep my feet up while I'm writing.

My breasts hurt a little, but I have no nausea, and the spotting continues. Six weeks and four days into the pregnancy—which is only about two weeks from the pregnancy test—I start bleeding more seriously and cramping. I call the fertility clinic the next morning, and they get me in for an ultrasound.

Everything is different at the clinic. We're all wearing masks and using hand sanitizer. The clinic is only half-staffed. The doctor who sees me—who is not a doctor I've ever met before—confirms that the bleeding is from another subchorionic hematoma. But, the baby measures the size he should, and there's a fetal heartbeat. The doctor is unconcerned about the bleeding and tells me lots of women at the clinic bleed. He seems to think this pregnancy is going to be fine.

That's not the big news, though. The big news is that the fertility clinic is closing. They're kicking me out. Or, as they put it, they're "graduating" me to a regular ob/gyn. But I'm being "graduated" a lot earlier than I was in the fall with that pregnancy, and it's happening even though I'm bleeding. I know this is because of Covid-19, but I still feel betrayed.

I continue to bleed, and I'm extremely tired, but the next week, I call the ob/gyn to set up my first appointment, and when I tell them I'm bleeding, the ob wants me to come in that day. On April 22, 2020, I see an obstetrician for this pregnancy for the first time.

I expect the baby to be dead. That's what I'm used to at visits like this. My expectations are not met. There is a visible subchorionic hematoma, but the baby is still there, he's still growing like he's supposed to, and his heartbeat is 142 beats per minute. They call what's happening to me a "threatened miscarriage," but the doctor says that's just insurance terminology. The pregnancy seems to be going well. They say, "try not to worry," and tell me to come back the next week.

Two days later, the bleeding seems to have stopped. I feel like maybe I'm in the clear. I sign up for a virtual paint night as a kind of celebration. So it makes perfect sense that at the end of virtual paint night, I stand up and gush blood. It's a good thing I'm at home, because the blood soaks my underwear and bleeds into my jeans. I run to the bathroom and drip bright red blood all over the tile. I have painful cramps along with the bleeding.

I have had so much bleeding by now that I know not to panic. I don't call the doctor or go to the hospital because the bleeding slows throughout the night and into the weekend, and for me, that means there's no reason for an ER visit. The baby is gone or not, but it's out of my control. I try to assume he's okay. (It's a little boy.) I worry anyway. I don't think bleeding during pregnancy ever makes a woman feel good.

I'm more exhausted than ever, maybe from the stress or from the progesterone shots I'm still taking or from the bleeding. By the end of the weekend, I have a bad migraine headache. The headache lasts until my next doctor's appointment on Tuesday. The bleeding is significantly lighter at that point, though, and the doctor tells us it looks like one of the clots has resolved. This should give me some comfort, but it doesn't. It's only week eight. My last pregnancy didn't end until week ten. Plus, I still don't have any morning sickness. Why not? I'm convinced that this is going to end in a miscarriage.

At our next appointment, I'm nine weeks, five days pregnant and expecting this to be the appointment where the doctor tells us the baby is gone. It's not. This is the one appointment in our whole pregnancy that goes completely well. The baby measures about an inch, his heart rate is 192 beats per minute, and we can see him wiggle! The hematoma is still visible on the ultrasound, but it's small and gray, and the doctor thinks this means it has clotted up and is absorbing into my body.

Malcolm and I are incredibly anxious, but the doctor tries to assure us that everything is fine. "This is a *normal* ultrasound," she tells us. "Everything we're seeing here is normal. You can stop being stressed out. The baby is doing great."

I get to stop taking the progesterone shots this week. I start to have energy again! Despite all the hope we'd lost, we now feel we can expect our pregnancy to be a routine pregnancy. We take a trip to a furniture store—with masks and gloves on—and for the first time, we feel genuinely optimistic. This baby is going to make it.

Our parents already know, and they're starting to get excited, too. We're thinking about when we might announce the pregnancy. I want to wait until the end of the first trimester, but that's only a couple of weeks away. I figure that we will be in the clear if we do it on week fourteen.

We feel happy for a few days.

NOTHING HURTS LIKE THIS

On May 21, 2020, we go to the doctor's office for our next appointment. I'm now eleven weeks, four days pregnant, so we're nearing the end of the first trimester.

I'm feeling far less fatigued, but I'm anxious again. I'm anxious at every appointment. We've had too much go wrong for me to kick that anxiety. Also, I can't feel anything happening inside, and I have no bump. A miscarriage could still happen. There's still reason to fear.

We have a different doctor at the ob/gyn office today. That's not a problem in itself—this office purposely tries to rotate pregnant women through all the doctors so that you don't have to deliver with someone you've never met at the end of your pregnancy. However, with the masks we're all wearing now and the fact that we've never met this doctor before, we have difficulty reading the doctor's facial expressions. That matters today, because the doctor doesn't seem happy during the ultrasound.

"His heart is beating, right?" I ask. "Is something wrong?"

The heart *is* beating—I haven't miscarried!—but the doctor still seems grim. He tells us he has noticed what he thinks is slightly thickened fluid behind the baby's neck. He wants us to see a genetic counselor because this can be a sign of Down Syndrome.

We don't understand. We had genetic testing done on this embryo. It's not supposed to be *possible* for our baby to be a Down's baby. The doctor explains that preimplantation genetic testing can be wrong. It's possible for the cells in an embryo to be different from each other at a chromosomal level. This is called mosaicism.

"But it's unlikely, and this could also be a sign of a heart defect," the doctor says. That makes me feel better. I was born with a little heart defect. Heart defects are fixable. I assume the referral to a genetic counselor is just a precaution. The doctor doesn't seem to share my relief, but again, we can't read his face. Maybe he's generally grumpy. Some doctors are.

He also mentions that the umbilical cord looks somewhat enlarged. Usually, this is something that goes away, he tells us, and he says the genetic counselor can talk to us more about it. It's the neck fluid he's concerned about. He tells us we should be getting a call to make an appointment with the genetic counselor soon, and we leave the office.

Malcolm and I talk nervously about this in the car on the way home. "It can't be Down's," I say. "We did genetic testing. That would be so freak."

Malcolm agrees. "And the doctor thinks it's not Down's. But then why did he seem so pessimistic?"

I try not to worry. We're "advanced maternal age." They probably refer everyone our age to a genetic counselor for even the slightest little problem.

But we get a call from a receptionist at a different office only an hour after we leave our ob/gyn. As it turns out, this *wasn't* just a referral to a genetic counselor. Our ob referred us to a doctor's office that specializes in high-risk pregnancies. This office wants to do their own ultrasound, then we'll talk to both a genetic counselor *and* a maternal-fetal specialist (MFM), a specialized ob/gyn that deals with high-risk pregnancies. They have an appointment available at 1pm this afternoon. Can we make it in today?

It is *never* good to get a same-day appointment because of a referral. So now we're really scared. We drop everything and drive to the new doctor's office, where a friendly ultrasound technician sees us. The baby's heart is beating so clearly, and we can see him wiggling all around in there. He must be fine, right? How can he be so active and not be fine?

The ultrasound technician can't tell us anything, so we try to take some comfort in what we see. We'll have to wait for the doctor to give us real results.

We're taken to a conference room where we wait while the maternal-fetal specialist doctor (the MFM) reviews the ultrasound pictures. Soon, the MFM comes into the room, along with a genetic counselor. They introduce themselves.

The doctor sits down. She says, "First, congratulations. It's a big deal to get this far."

Okay. So far so good.

Then she asks us to tell her what our ob told us this morning. We repeat what our ob told us about Down's and a potential heart defect.

The doctor says, "We do not appreciate any increased fluid around the neck."

It takes me a minute to understand what she means by that. She doesn't "appreciate" it? Like, she doesn't appreciate that the ob even mentioned it or something? We ask for some clarification. She means that this clinic doesn't see what he saw. There is no increased fluid that would indicate Down Syndrome.

This is a huge relief. I feel like I can breathe easier. For five seconds. Because after that, the doctor goes on to tell us that what they *do* see are a single umbilical artery cord and an omphalocele.

A what and a what?

She says the umbilical cord is supposed to have two arteries. Our baby's umbilical cord only has one. That is called a single umbilical artery. It is fairly common and doesn't always create an issue, but in our case, it comes with an omphalocele, which is a far rarer and more serious issue.

The doctor explains that an embryo's abdominal organs are developing outside its body between weeks eight and ten. Normally, during that time, the baby folds up around itself like a pancake folding up, which encloses the baby's organs inside its body.

An omphalocele is what happens when the baby's tummy doesn't completely close up. Instead, some of the baby's abdominal organs stay outside the body and grow in a little sac where the umbilical cord meets the baby's stomach.

The doctor says it is a rare abdominal defect, and although omphaloceles sometimes resolve, our baby's omphalocele appears too big to resolve. In the majority of these cases, an omphalocele is related to a major chromosomal abnormality or some other major genetic disorder. It's not typically Down's, though. Our baby is more likely to be a Trisomy 13 or Trisomy 18 baby, which is *much* worse because Trisomy 13 and Trisomy 18 babies don't typically survive to birth. If they do survive, they hardly ever live longer than a year.

The genetic counselor tries to explain this further to us after the doctor says her bit, and the counselor suggests additional genetic screening. There's a blood test we can do today that would serve as a second genetic screening test (the preimplantation genetic testing we did was the first), and we should have the results back in a week. The word "termination" is brought up, and we learn that in North Carolina, we only have until week twenty to terminate. Virginia, which is a three-hour drive from us, would allow us slightly more time.

Termination.

They're talking about us terminating a baby we've waited almost a decade for because he could have such a bad chromosomal abnormality that he would only suffer if he even managed to survive to birth.

"But what if his chromosomes are normal?" I ask.

The doctor tells us that if there aren't other problems and the omphalocele is "isolated," then it's often possible to surgically correct an omphalocele. But that's especially rare. Usually, even if there aren't chromosomal abnormalities, there are other major problems. Also, the surgical correction can't happen until after birth, and we're a long way from even having that discussion.

The doctor asks us to schedule a follow-up appointment in two weeks. They'll look at the omphalocele again at that point to confirm the diagnosis, and they will talk to us about the genetic screening results.

Malcolm and I have an awful weekend. We cry. We pray. We Google everything. We hope that maybe the omphalocele will resolve. Maybe the doctor was wrong. Maybe the omphalocele isn't that big. Thankfully, we get the genetic screening results back at the end of the week and learn that the results are normal. This is a big win. Surely it means the omphalocele will resolve? Surely this won't kill the baby?

But when we go back for an appointment on June 4, the omphalocele is still there. We have another MFM this time, and he says it is a "very large" omphalocele. He sounds downright pessimistic. He tells us the omphalocele isn't going to resolve.

Even though the genetic screening results came back normal, he recommends we do a chorionic villus sampling (CVS) test. This will allow the doctor to collect sample DNA that will be sent to a lab for diagnostic genetic testing. Genetic testing, it turns out, is not all created equal. We spend an hour with a genetic counselor trying to understand how the two genetic screening tests we've already done could be wrong. We learn that there *are* reasons a screening test may not detect something that a diagnostic test could. Despite our two normal tests, the baby's chromosomes still might not be normal.

We schedule the CVS test for the next day, then we wait for those results. It should only take ten business days for the results to come back, but in our case, the sample cells grow too slowly for that. We get a call from the genetic counselor letting us know that our results may take three or four weeks.

In the meanwhile, we return to the doctor's office for another appointment. We are now at week sixteen of the pregnancy. The doctor comes into the room after the ultrasound scan, sits down, and says, "I'm disappointed by these results." He tells us that in addition to a very large omphalocele, the baby also has short long bones, scoliosis, and evidence of a heart defect.

He is *sure* the genetic test results are going to show an abnormality of some kind. Even if the baby doesn't have a large problem like Trisomy 13 or Trisomy 18, he could still have a microdeletion or some other smaller chromosomal abnormality.

These smaller abnormalities are very serious. The doctor tells us they would still mean a significantly increased risk of fetal death (a stillborn baby). If the baby survives and we try to correct any of the problems, we will likely be making a baby who might not even live "suffer" (the doctor's word) through a lot of surgery for nothing. If the baby makes it through that kind of surgery, he will have major developmental delays.

If we want to consider termination, we need to decide by week eighteen of the pregnancy so that they can get us an operating room for the procedure in time for the North Carolina abortion cut off.

We do not *want* to terminate our baby, and we also do not want to make our baby suffer. Furthermore, we don't have the information we need to make any choice yet. The baby's genetic testing isn't back—the doctor could be wrong—but even if we get the results back by week eighteen, there could be other problems. If the baby has a major heart defect, that would also mean a high risk of a stillbirth or a baby that might not survive, and it's too early now for an ultrasound to accurately show a heart defect.

This is not an unplanned pregnancy. This is not an unwanted baby. We want to fight for this baby and give him as much time as possible. But thanks to that strict legal cut-off, our doctor is talking to us about termination and we are in a position where we might need to make a decision before we know if the baby stands a chance. We're stunned that a law we never expected to apply to us is now putting pressure on us to terminate a baby we desperately want. Why on earth isn't there at least an exception to the termination cut-off for a baby who has a major birth defect that could kill him or make him suffer if he is born?

The doctor does give us another path, though. If we don't want to terminate, we can opt to try to have the baby and choose palliative care after birth. Meaning, we could wait and see if the baby survives to birth, praying that the baby doesn't suffer dying in the womb. Then, after the baby is born, we can put him straight into hospice. The baby would be given pain relief and comfort care but would not have to endure any surgery. We would be with him while he died.

Those are the three pathways the doctor gives us. (A) Termination. (B) Surgery and suffering. (C) Wait and palliative care. The doctor's report later says "poor prognosis."

I don't ever remember feeling sadder in my life.

COUNT YOUR BLESSINGS

You know what, though? I really am a whole hell of a lot stronger than I think. I'm far stronger than I was before my infertility journey started. So is Malcolm.

Despite those terrible appointments, neither of us fall

apart. We hold out for those diagnostic genetic testing results. We cry, but we are kind to each other. Malcolm continues to distract himself with work. I'm having trouble concentrating, but I still get up every day, shower, and work on my writing as much as I can. We pray. A lot.

I'm grateful to be on a depression medication (and no, I am not on a medication that would have caused the omphalocele). I'm grateful to have a therapist for stress management help already. I finish another novella I've been working on despite all the stress, and I publish it. I think it's one of my favorites.

Then, finally, some hope appears. We get the diagnostic genetic testing results back. The baby does *not* have any chromosomal abnormalities. He could still have a smaller genetic problem, but he might be perfectly normal other than the omphalocele. He's not a Trisomy 13 or 18 baby. He doesn't have microdeletions or translocations in his chromosomes.

At week eighteen, we go to a pediatric cardiologist for a fetal echocardiogram. That's a specialized ultrasound to look specifically at the potential heart defect our MFM is concerned about. The pediatric cardiologist gives us more good news. There is no heart defect. The baby's heart is tilted a little left, but that's probably because an omphalocele can cause some displacement of organs. The cardiologist says this is not likely to be an issue for the baby, it's not something to surgically correct, and he doesn't see anything wrong with the baby's heart. He doesn't expect to see us again for the rest of the pregnancy.

We have a comprehensive anatomy scan done at week twenty-one. We see a third MFM that day from the same high-risk pregnancy clinic, and we do this purposefully so that we can get another set of eyes on the baby. The baby does have a large omphalocele. The doctors expect it to be classified as a "giant" omphalocele by the time he's born. He also measures small, but this, the MFM says, is probably because fetal measurements are based on abdominal circumference measurements, and an omphalocele makes those measurements difficult to take accurately.

Given the genetic testing results and the results of the fetal echocardiogram, the MFM thinks we should plan for a week thirty-nine C-section. After that, the baby will need surgery. The doctor warns us that this surgery might not happen immediately after birth. The baby could be in the Neonatal Intensive Care Unit (NICU) for a while before we can take him home.

"But what are our chances that he'll be stillborn?" I ask.

The doctor tells us she thinks those chances are low. She thinks he'll survive to birth. It's week twenty-one, and we've been dealing with this terrifying diagnosis since week eleven. It took that long for us to finally reach the point where our doctors think *the baby might survive and live a healthy life.*

The doctors stop talking about termination, suffering, and palliative care. Everyone seems more positive now, and when we start talking to the doctors who are going to be taking care of our baby after he's born, there's even more optimism.

The NICU doctors want us to expect that the baby will spend a few months in NICU after he's born, and they tell me to prepare to give birth a little earlier than week thirty-nine if necessary, because that might happen with this baby. Since the baby has a giant omphalocele, there are possible complications to worry about.

Nothing about this will be easy, but the prognosis is no longer "poor." We don't need the baby to be "fixed" immediately. We can be patient with whatever he needs. He'll be perfect to us if he just lives and doesn't suffer.

The pediatric surgeon is the most optimistic of the doctors we speak with. She tells us that if there aren't other issues that come up, the baby's likelihood of survival is probably 90% or more.

90% or more.

The baby has a real fighting chance.

I cry every time I think about that.

NOT OVER YET

As I publish this book, I am thirty-eight weeks pregnant, and there is only one week before our scheduled C-section.

Malcolm is still working from home thanks to Covid-19. Ruth Bader Ginsberg and Alex Trebek both died this fall. Our favorite wineries in California are all at risk of burning down. The presidential election is over, but President Trump refuses to concede that Joe Biden won.

We've tried to prepare for the birth of our baby as much as possible. We have hospital bags already packed. We've rented an AirBnB for most of December so that we can be as close to the NICU as possible immediately after our baby is born, even though the hospital is only a thirty-minute drive from our house. We have barely been anywhere since February because it's that important to us not to get covid.

We still have no guarantees. We do not know if the baby will be okay. We do not know how this story ends. We don't even know if our infertility journey is finally over. It's possible that it's not. There's still one more embryo left—a girl—and if we've learned anything from our infertility experience, it's that there's no sense in expecting that you can control or plan anything related to making a baby.

Babies are miracles.

The baby I'm carrying right now is an incredible, amazing, awesome miracle. That is the only thing I can tell you for sure about him.

I can, however, tell you a few more things about myself. I can tell you I'm more resilient than I thought I was. I'm braver. I'm more capable, more confident, more patient, more creative. I can make it through physical and emotional pain. I can survive things I didn't think I could survive. I can survive the unexpected. I've accomplished things I didn't think I could. I'm tougher than ever. I have stories to tell.

My marriage is stronger than I thought, too, and my husband is stronger and more resilient, and he can handle difficult things. We are hard workers who have great friends and loving families. We've shared amazing adventures and amazing bottles of wine. We're better all the time at loving and supporting each other. It's a work in progress, but there *is* continual progress.

And none of this happened because our thirties were easy. This happened because we had a difficult infertility journey that isn't even over yet.

For some people, difficulties create trauma and fear. Bad times give them reasons to be triggered and to shut down. Maybe it's my personality, my perspective, or the way I was raised, or maybe it's because I write young adult fantasy fiction and I believe in the "hero's journey," but I'm not like that. For me, making it through one challenge is a reason to believe I can make it through another, harder challenge.

I didn't share my story because I want you to see all the ways infertility has destroyed me over the years. I also didn't share it to sensationalize infertility or scare you. I promise you, giant omphaloceles are incredibly rare. Rare, like, 1 in 10,000. 1 in 9 women have trouble getting pregnant. It's far more likely for you to need IVF than for you to ever have a doctor tell you your unborn baby has a "poor prognosis."

You shouldn't take from this that you're in for an awful time if you have to face your own infertility journey. I shared my story because I wanted to give anyone going through this a fair and realistic look at what infertility truly entails.

At times it is gory, painful, embarrassing, frustrating, and devastating. It will defy your expectations, shatter your dreams, cause you grief and loss. You will see your relationships change because of it. You will see your life change.

Your own journey may be easier than mine. It also may be more difficult than mine. You'll wish you had a crystal ball, but there will be no way to predict how this ends for you. I still don't know how this ends for me, and I have a C-section planned for next week.

But despite all that, there's good news. This doesn't have to be a tragedy for you. You can let infertility change you for the better. You can let this grow your life in beautiful ways. Your odds of survival are high, even if you're in this storm for a very long time.

I'm still surviving. Maybe I'm even thriving.

And as for the rest of my story? Stay tuned. When I learn how to navigate the NICU and be the mom of a child who needs extra special care, I'll let you know. I hear it's not quite the same as what you expect when you're expecting.

Then again, I hear some people just have sex if they want to have a baby. I'm used to the unexpected. Let's see what comes next.

The end. For now.

PART VII

Appendices & Endnotes

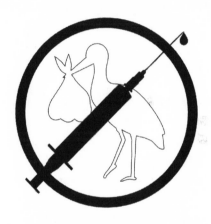

Here you will find all the extra stuff I thought
you might want after reading this book.

~ Me

APPENDIX A: GLOSSARY
Infertility Lingo

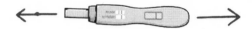

WHAT'S THIS?

This glossary includes terminology and definitions that relate to my infertility journey specifically. Other infertility procedures, conditions, tests, and treatments do exist.

CONDITIONS THAT CAUSE INFERTILITY

Adenomyosis. A condition where the endometrial tissue lining the inside of the uterine wall grows into the outer muscular walls of the uterus, causing the uterus to thicken and enlarge.[68]

Endometriosis. A condition where the endometrium, which is the inner lining of the uterus, develops in places other than the inner lining of the uterus, such as on the ovaries or on the fallopian tubes.[69]

Polycystic Ovarian Syndrome (PCOS). A disorder where women have infrequent or long menstrual periods or excess male hormone levels. Women with PCOS often develop small follicles on their ovaries, but they do not regularly ovulate (release eggs).[70]

HORMONES RELATED TO INFERTILITY.

Follicle-stimulating hormone (FSH). A hormone made by your pituitary gland that makes the follicles on your ovaries grow. A follicle is a small cyst that contains an egg. Your FSH levels start low at the beginning of your cycle, then go up, causing a follicle to grow and the egg to mature. FSH is usually tested between day 1 and 5 of your cycle.[71]

Estradiol. A hormone that tells the pituitary gland it doesn't need to make as much FSH. Estradiol is also tested early in your cycle. It's supposed to be low at the beginning.[72]

Antimüllerian hormone (AMH). A hormone made in the follicle and related to the number of eggs you have left (your "ovarian reserve"). It can be tested any time during your menstrual cycle.[73]

Progesterone. A hormone that helps a woman's uterus prepare for and maintain a pregnancy by thickening the lining of the uterus.[74] It is often tested throughout your cycle.

Thyroid-stimulating hormone (TSH). A hormone produced by the thyroid gland, which makes all kinds of hormones that regulate your body's use of energy in many complicated ways.[75] Low levels of TSH can prevent your body from properly releasing eggs.[76]

GENETIC TESTING

Carrier screening. Genetic testing done to determine whether you carry genes for specific genetic disorders, such as cystic fibrosis, hemoglobinopathies, spinal muscular atrophy (SMA), fragile X syndrome, sickle cell disease, and Tay–Sachs disease.[77] Usually, this screening only requires a blood, saliva, or tissue sample.

Preimplantation Genetic Testing (PGT). Genetic testing of embryos. To perform the testing, a tiny sample is taken from a frozen embryo and sent to a lab that cultures the sample (i.e. grows it). The lab can then perform Preimplantation Genetic Screening (PGS) to test the sample for chromosomal abnormalities. The lab may also perform Preimplantation Genetic Diagnosis (PGD) to test the sample for a specific, known genetic mutation.[78]

DIAGNOSTIC INFERTILITY TESTING

Pelvic ultrasound. A procedure where a "transducer" (the ultrasound wand) is used to send out ultrasound waves that move within the body to the organs and structures inside. The sound then bounces off those organs like an echo, the transducer processes the echoes, and those are converted into images of the organs and structures being examined.

A pelvic ultrasound can be done transabdominally

(transducer wand and gel are placed on your belly) or transvaginally (wand and gel are inserted into your vagina).[79]

Saline infusion sonohysterography (SIS or SHG) (the "saline ultrasound"). A procedure where sterile fluid is pumped into your uterus through your cervix and then an ultrasound is performed so the doctor can check your uterus, uterine lining, and ovaries for abnormalities.[80]

Hysterosalpingogram (HSG). A procedure where iodine is pumped into your uterus through your cervix and then an x-ray is performed so the doctor can check to see whether your fallopian tubes are open and whether your uterus is normal.[81]

Hysteroscopy. A procedure where the cervix is stretched so that a hysteroscope (which looks like a very long needle and is sort of like a telescope) can be threaded through your cervix and into your uterus. The hysteroscope can then be used to give your doctor a better look at your uterus or to allow your doctor to do things like remove scar tissue from the inside of your uterus. A hysteroscopy can be performed in a physician's office or in an operating room.[82]

Mock Embryo Cycle with Uterine Biopsy for Endometrial Receptivity Analysis (ERA). An ERA is a genetic test where a sample of a woman's endometrial lining is analyzed to determine what the best day is to transfer an embryo during an IVF cycle. To obtain the sample, you goes through a "mock" embryo transfer cycle, taking all the same medications you would take and/or inject for a real IVF cycle, but instead of transferring an embryo to your uterus when your uterus is ready, an endometrial biopsy is performed instead, where the doctor snips out a sample of your uterus lining to send to a lab for testing.[83]

INFERTILITY TREATMENTS

Timed Intercourse. A low-intervention infertility treatment option where a woman's cycle is closely monitored to detect ovulation and the woman has sex with her partner soon before and during ovulation. This is sometimes done with drugs to stimulate ovulation, such as Clomiphene Citrate (Clomid) or Letrozole (Femara).[84]

Intrauterine Insemination (IUI). A procedure where sperm is injected into a woman's uterus while she is ovulating. Sperm is collected from the woman's partner in advance or donated. In an IUI cycle, the woman often takes drugs such as Clomiphene Citrate (Clomid) or Letrozle (Femara) to stimulate ovulation before the procedure.[85]

In Vitro Fertilization (IVF). A procedure where an egg is combined with sperm in the hopes that the egg will be fertilized and result in an embryo. The embryo is then transferred to a woman's uterus, where it may implant, impregnating the woman.[86] IVF can be done with a "fresh" embryo or a "frozen" embryo.[87]

"Fresh" IVF Cycle. In the case of a "fresh" embryo transfer, the IVF cycle involves two procedures. First, the woman's ovaries are stimulated with medication to produce eggs, then eggs are surgically "retrieved" and combined with sperm for fertilization in a laboratory. Second, an embryo created during this process is transferred back into the woman three or five days after the retrieval.

"Frozen" IVF Cycle. In the case of a "frozen" embryo transfer, there is no ovarian stimulation or egg retrieval involved in the IVF cycle. Instead, an embryo that was previously created from a fresh cycle and then frozen is thawed and transferred back into the woman. These are also called "FET" cycles.

Intracytoplasmic Sperm Injection (ICSI). Sometimes sperm need help penetrating the outer layer of an egg for whatever reason during the fertilization process, so instead of just combining egg and sperm in lab dishes, a procedure is done where a single sperm is injected directly into the egg.[88]

PREGNANCY LOSS

Miscarriage. When an baby dies before the 20th week of pregnancy.[89]

Stillbirth. When a baby is lost (fetal death) after the 20th week of pregnancy.[90]

Dilation and curettage (D&C). A procedure to remove tissue from your uterus. This is often done after a miscarriage or abortion or to treat a condition like heavy bleeding.[91]

APPENDIX B: TIME & MONEY
A Chronology of Our Treatments

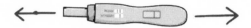

WHAT'S THIS?

This is a chronology of all our infertility treatments, including information about how long things took and what it all cost. Spoiler alert: it took a long time and cost a lot of money.

DECEMBER 2011
Age: 30

We live together in downtown Chicago with our dog, who is still a puppy. We get married at Fourth Presbyterian Church. We look so young in the pictures. I am on birth control. My skin looks great.

SPRING/FALL 2012
Age: 30

I am going through a depression, and I am worried about my fertility. In the spring, at my annual ob/gyn appointment, I ask my gynecologist about metformin. She says it won't help me. I'm frustrated. I stop taking birth control anyway. We do not use condoms. I hope to get pregnant but know it is unlikely. I track my basal body temperature. I do not start getting periods.

By fall, I'm desperate for something that will restore my periods. I make another appointment with my gynecologist to talk specifically about metformin again. This time my doctor reluctantly prescribes the metformin but repeats that it won't help me and could have ugly side effects.

I do not experience any bad side effects. I do start losing a little weight. I continue to track my basal body temperature on and off. I still do not start getting periods.

SPRING/SUMMER 2013
Age: 31

I continue to lose weight, but my periods don't start, and by the time my next annual ob/gyn appointment rolls around, my skin is breaking out and I'm losing hair. I ask my gynecologist to put me back on birth control.

By summer, I am down two sizes from what I weighed when I got married. Malcolm and I move to Marietta, Georgia. I go off birth control again, and we start actively trying to get pregnant. I still don't get periods, and I do not get pregnant.

SPRING/SUMMER 2014
Age: 32

We have our first consult with a local fertility clinic. We do carrier screening, a semen analysis, a saline ultrasound, and an HSG test. Then we start our first infertility treatment cycles. We do three cycles. None result in a pregnancy.

Cycle 1: Timed Intercourse with Clomid
Pregnancy test result: negative
Cost: $1,953

Cycle 2: IUI with Clomid
Pregnancy test result: negative
Cost: $2,272

Cycle 3: IUI with Clomid
Pregnancy test result: negative
Cost: $2,646

Total No. of Cycles: 3
Total Time: 5 months
Total Cost: $6,871

FALL 2014-SPRING 2015
Age: 33

We go back to the doctor for a consult, he does another saline ultrasound and a diagnostic hysteroscopy. Then we do a fresh IVF cycle with semen collection, egg stimulation, egg retrieval, embryo transfer, and a pregnancy test. I get pregnant but later miscarry. I undergo a D&C.

Cycle 4: Fresh IVF
Embryos transferred: 1
Pregnancy test result: positive, then miscarriage
Cost: $235 for the consult, $13,125 for the IVF
cycle, $3,328 for diagnostic testing, semen collection, and prescription drugs, $719 for the D&C

Total No. of Cycles: 1
Total Time: 6 months
Total Cost: $17,407

SUMMER 2015 - SPRING 2017
Age: 33 - 35

I go through another bad depression, and we take what we think might be a "forever" break from infertility treatments. In the meanwhile, our fertility clinic is storing the two remaining embryos from our fresh IVF cycle. The cost of storage for two years is approximately $800.

Total No. of Cycles: 0
Total Time: 2 years
Total Cost: $800

SUMMER/FALL 2017
Age: 35

We return to the fertility clinic, though we switch doctors. We start IVF treatments again, first using the two frozen embryos we have left. When those two frozen cycles fail, our doctor recommends a "mock embryo transfer cycle" and Endometrial Receptivity Analysis.

After the mock cycle is over, we have the extra eggs we'd frozen after our fresh IVF cycle fertilized. This gives us two more embryos, which we transfer during one more frozen IVF cycle. We do not get any positive pregnancy tests.

IVF is covered by our insurance this year, but we have a high deductible plan, so we still have to pay a few thousand dollars. Also, some of the labs our fertility clinic works with are not "in network," so we have to submit some bills to our insurance company later for reimbursement. Because of these complications, the cost numbers below are estimates.

Cycle 5: Frozen IVF
Embryos transferred: 1
Pregnancy test result: negative

Cycle 6: Frozen IVF
Embryos transferred: 1
Pregnancy test result: negative

Cycle 7: Mock Embryo Cycle
No embryos transferred.
No pregnancy test.

Cycle 8: Frozen IVF
Embryos transferred: 2
Pregnancy test result: negative

Total No. of Cycles: 4
Total Time: 7 months
Total Cost: $3,340

SPRING 2018
Age: 36

Exhausted from IVF, we ask our doctor if there is any way we can go back to some low-key timed intercourse cycles. She helps us do that. Again, these cycles are basically covered by our insurance, but we have a high-deductible plan, so we still have to pay a portion of the costs out of pocket.

Cycle 9: Timed Intercourse
(No drugs! I'm randomly ovulating!)
Pregnancy test result: negative

Cycle 10: Timed Intercourse with Clomid
Pregnancy test result: negative

Cycle 11: Timed Intercourse with Clomid
Pregnancy test result: negative

Total No. of Cycles: 3
Total Time: 4 months
Total Cost: $1,214

SUMMER/FALL 2018
Age: 36-37

We move again, this time to Raleigh, North Carolina, and find a new fertility clinic and a new doctor.

We schedule a consult with the doctor, and he recommends an egg retrieval cycle with genetic testing of the embryos. We get 10 embryos from the egg retrieval cycle, and we send samples of all those embryos for genetic screening. Of the 10 embryos, only 4 are normal. The other 6 have chromosomal abnormalities and are discarded.

Our insurance covers some diagnostic tests and some meds, but otherwise, we must pay out of pocket.

Cycle 12: Egg Retrieval & Genetic Screening

No embryos transferred.

No pregnancy test.

Cost: $60 for the consults, $15,625 for the egg retrieval, monitoring appointments, and frozen cycle (which we did later), $4,312 for the medications, $1,550 for the genetic screening

Total No. of Cycles: 1
Total Time: 4 months
Total Cost: $21,547

2019

Age: 37

We begin the year by paying a storage fee of $525 to the fertility clinic for our four frozen embryos. Then, before we can start a frozen cycle with any of those frozen embryos, the doctor recommends diagnostic testing. We do a saline ultrasound, a second mock embryo cycle with ERA, a diagnostic hysteroscopy, and a pelvic MRI.

The doctor diagnoses me with adenomyosis and recommends a three-month course of Lupron Depot shots to reduce the size of my uterus and prepare it for IVF. We then proceed with our first frozen IVF cycle with this clinic.

The pregnancy test is negative. We move on to a second frozen IVF cycle fairly quickly, and that cycle results in a positive pregnancy test. We are thrilled, but there are challenges. I bleed a lot in my first trimester thanks to some subchorionic hematomas. In November, ten weeks into the pregnancy, we learn that we have lost the baby. I go through another D&C.

Cycle 13: Mock Embryo Cycle + Diagnostic Testing + Lupron Depot Shots
No embryos transferred.
No pregnancy test.
Cost: $2,522 for the tests, $266 for the shots

Cycle 14: Frozen IVF
Embryos transferred: 1
Pregnancy test result: negative
Cost: $55 for the scheduling class, $15 for the meds, $525 for embryo storage
(We had pre-paid for most of this cycle with the egg retrieval cycle.)

Cycle 15: Frozen IVF
Embryos transferred: 1
Pregnancy test result: positive, then miscarriage
Cost: $4,149 for the frozen IVF cycle, $165 for the meds, $96 for ultrasounds after a pregnancy was confirmed, $444 for the D&C and follow-up.

Total No. of Cycles: 3
Total Time: 11 months
Total Cost: $8,237

2020

Age: 38

We begin the year again by paying a storage fee of $525 to the fertility clinic for our remaining two frozen embryos. We are not optimistic about our third frozen IVF cycle with this clinic. Also, as always, there are tests to be done before we can get started. In January, we do a saline ultrasound and then another hysteroscopy.

In February, we do our third frozen IVF cycle with this clinic. The embryo transfer takes place on March 20, 2020, only a week after the World Health Organization declares Covid-19 a global pandemic.

The pregnancy test is positive, but I bleed again from subchorionic hematomas. We "graduate" from the fertility clinic to a regular ob/gyn. Throughout the entire first trimester, I am terrified of losing the baby.

On May 21, 2020, at a routine, week eleven appointment, our ob notices something abnormal on our ultrasound. We are seen the same day by a maternal-fetal medicine (MFM) specialist at a high-risk pregnancy clinic.

The doctor and a genetic counselor sit us down in a conference room and tell us our baby has a single umbilical artery and an omphalocele, which is a major abdominal wall defect that is extremely likely to indicate a chromosomal abnormality. They talk to us about termination and additional genetic testing.

We spend the next several weeks in testing limbo. We do not breathe a sigh of relief until the end of June, when we finally learn that the baby does not have any chromosomal abnormalities and also does not appear to have other major birth defects.

The baby has what will probably be classified as a "giant omphalocele" and will need serious surgery after birth. There could be major complications, but the baby has a high chance of survival. We pray a lot.

Cycle 16: Frozen IVF
Embryos transferred: 1
Pregnancy test result: positive
Cost: $525 for embryo storage, $671 for tests, $4,000 for the IVF Cycle, $224 for meds, $30 for ultrasound at fertility clinic after pregnancy was confirmed, and then …?
(We do not have a total yet for how much money
we paid to our regular ob/gyn and then our MFM
for continuing pregnancy monitoring.)

Total No. of Cycles: 1
Total Time (to date): 11 months
Total Costs: $5,450

PRESENT DAY
Age: 39

As of this book's publication, the baby has not yet been born, thus the ambiguous ending. We are enormously grateful to have built up enough strength over the last decade to be able to withstand what has been an incredibly challenging pregnancy.

<u>ALL-TIME TOTALS</u>

Years Spent Trying to Have a Baby: 8 Years, 8 Months
Infertility Treatment Cycles: 16
Fertility Clinics: 2
Reproductive Endocrinologists: 3
Timed Intercourse / IUI Cycles: 6
IVF/Egg Retrieval/Mock Cycles: 10

Pregnancy Tests: 13
Pregnancies: 3
Miscarriages: 2

Total Costs: $64,866

Live Births: Hopefully 1
But we know all babies are miracles and there
are no guarantees. We continue to pray.

APPENDIX C : ADDITIONAL RESOURCES
Useful Sources of Information

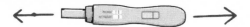

INFERTILITY ORGANIZATIONS

1. American Society for Reproductive Medicine (ASRM)
https://www.reproductivefacts.org/

Lots of information about what various
infertility terms and treatments mean.

2. Society for Assisted Reproductive Technology (SART)
https://sart.org/

Statistics on IVF success rates.
Information about your local clinic.

3. Resolve: The National Infertility Association
https://resolve.org/

Advocacy.

BOOKS I FOUND HELPFUL

1. *Taking Charge of Your Fertility, 20th Anniversary Edition: The Definitive Guide to Natural Birth Control, Pregnancy Achievement, and Reproductive Health* by Toni Weschler

The classic "how to deal with infertility book." For people who want to learn comprehensive information about their reproductive system and why it might not be working.

2. *Infreakinfertility: How to Survive When Getting Pregnant Gets Hard* by Melanie Dale

A hilarious take on infertility from another woman who learned how to survive it.

3. *It's OK That You're Not OK: Meeting Grief and Loss in a Culture That Doesn't Understand* by Megan Devine

The book that made me feel better about my grief after my miscarriages.

4. *The Body Keeps the Score: Brain, Mind, and Body in the Healing of Trauma* by Bessel van der Kolk M.D.

In case you think that the emotional pain of infertility will in no way affect your physical health.

5. *The Gifts of Imperfection: Let Go of Who You Think You're Suppose♦ to Be an♦ Embrace Who You Are* by Brené Brown

For anyone who can't handle the whole "you can't control this" thing about infertility.

6. *Ra♦ical Acceptance: Embracing Your Life With the Heart of a Bu♦♦ha* by Tara Brach

For getting "zen" about life challenges.

7. *Big Magic: Creative Living Beyon♦ Fear* by Elizabeth Gilbert

Because your legacy needs to be something beyond having babies.

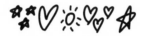

ENDNOTES
Fact Check My Facts

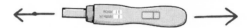

1   "Age and Fertility," American Society for Reproductive
    Medicine, last updated 2012, https://www.reproductivefacts.
    org/news-and-publications/patient-fact-sheets-and-booklets/
    documents/fact-sheets-and-info-booklets/age-and-fertility/.
2   Sanoff, Rachel, "How to Make Sex Ed Better in America," *Bustle*,
    August 27, 2015, https://www.bustle.com/articles/104233-7-
    problems-with-the-state-of-sex-ed-in-america-today-and-how-
    we-can-make.
3   "How to Get Pregnant," Tommy's, last reviewed on June 5th,
    2018, last accessed October 31, 2020, https://www.tommys.
    org/pregnancy-information/planning-pregnancy/how-get-
    pregnant; Corinna, Heather with Isabella Rotman, "Human
    Reproduction: A Seafarer's Guide," Scarleteen, last accessed
    October 8, 2020, https://www.scarleteen.com/article/bodies/
    where_did_i_come_from_a_refresher_course_in_human_
    reproduction; "How Pregnancy Happens," Planned Parenthood,
    last accessed October 8, 2020, https://www.plannedparenthood.
    org/learn/pregnancy/how-pregnancy-happens.
4   Firth, Shannon, "Study: Infertile Couples 3 Times More
    Likely to Divorce," U.S. News & World Report, January 30,
    2014, https://www.usnews.com/news/articles/2014/01/31/
    study-infertile-couples-3-times-more-likely-to-divorce.

5   Tao, Peng et al., "Investigating Marital Relationship in Infertility: A Systematic Review of Quantitative Studies," *Journal of Reproductive Infertility*, 13, 2 (2012): 71-80, https://www.ncbi.nlm.nih.gov/pmc/articles/PMC3719332/.

6   Millheiser, Leah S., M.D. et al., "Is Infertility a Risk Factor for Female Sexual Dysfunction? A Case-Control Study," *Fertility and Sterility*, 94, 6 (2010): 2022-2025, https://doi.org/10.1016/j.fertnstert.2010.01.037.

7   "Ovarian Reserve," American Society for Reproductive Medicine, revised 2014, https://www.reproductivefacts.org/news-and-publications/patient-fact-sheets-and-booklets/documents/fact-sheets-and-info-booklets/ovarian-reserve/.

8   "Carrier Screening," The American College of Obstetricians and Gynecologists, last accessed October 8, 2020, https://www.acog.org/patient-resources/faqs/pregnancy/carrier-screening.

9   Tobah, Yvonne Butler, M.D., "Hypothyroidism and Infertility: Any Connection?" Mayo Clinic (Blog), June 13, 2019, https://www.mayoclinic.org/diseases-conditions/female-infertility/expert-answers/hypothyroidism-and-infertility/faq-20058311.

10   "Saline Infusion Sonohysterogram (SHG)," American Society for Reproductive Medicine, revised 2015, https://www.reproductivefacts.org/news-and-publications/patient-fact-sheets-and-booklets/documents/fact-sheets-and-info-booklets/saline-infusion-sonohysterogram-shg/.

11   "Hysterosalpingogram (HSG)," American Society for Reproductive Medicine, revised 2015, https://www.reproductivefacts.org/news-and-publications/patient-fact-sheets-and-booklets/documents/fact-sheets-and-info-booklets/.

12   "Laparoscopy and Hysteroscopy," American Society for Reproductive Medicine, 2016, https://www.reproductivefacts.org/news-and-publications/patient-fact-sheets-and-booklets/documents/fact-sheets-and-info-booklets/laparoscopy-and-hysteroscopy-booklet/.

13   "What to Know About Endometrial Receptivity Analysis," Igenomix (blog), February 2, 2019,

https://www.igenomix.com/fertility-challenges/
what-to-know-about-endometrial-receptivity-analysis/.

14 Epel, E., Daubenmier, J., Moskowitz, J.T., Folkman, S. and Blackburn, E., "Can Meditation Slow Rate of Cellular Aging? Cognitive Stress, Mindfulness, and Telomeres." *Annals of the New York Academy of Sciences*, 1172 (2009): 34-53, https://doi.org/10.1111/j.1749-6632.2009.04414.x.

15 "Polycystic Ovary Syndrome (PCOS)," Mayo Clinic, last accessed October 8, 2020, https://www.mayoclinic.org/diseases-conditions/pcos/symptoms-causes/syc-20353439.

16 "Pelvic Ultrasound," Johns Hopkins Medicine, last accessed October 8, 2020, https://www.hopkinsmedicine.org/health/treatment-tests-and-therapies/pelvic-ultrasound.

17 "Fertility Drugs And The Risk of Multiple Births," American Society for Reproductive Health, revised 2012, https://www.reproductivefacts.org/news-and-publications/patient-fact-sheets-and-booklets/documents/fact-sheets-and-info-booklets/fertility-drugs-and-the-risk-of-multiple-births/.

18 "Having Healthy Babies One at a Time," Centers for Disease Control and Prevention, last accessed October 13, 2020, https://www.cdc.gov/art/pdf/patient-resources/Having-Healthy-Babies-handout-2_508tagged.pdf.

19 "Everything You Need to Know About Timed Intercourse," Fertility Center of Illinois (blog), November 13, 2019, https://www.fcionline.com/fertility-blog/everything-you-need-to-know-about-timed-intercourse.

20 "What is IUI?" Resolve, last accessed October 8, 2020, https://resolve.org/what-are-my-options/treatment-options/what-is-iui/.

21 Rodriguez, Tori, "Laugh Lots, Live Longer," *Scientific American Mind*, 27 (2016): 17, https://www.scientificamerican.com/article/laugh-lots-live-longer/.

22 "What is IVF?" Resolve, last accessed October 8, 2020, https://resolve.org/what-are-my-options/treatment-options/what-is-ivf/.

23 "Fresh and Frozen Embryo Transfers," Society for Assisted Reproductive Technology, last accessed October 8, 2020, https://www.sart.org/patients/fyi-videos/fresh-and-frozen-embryo-transfers/.

24 "Ovarian Hyperstimulation Syndrome," Mayo Clinic, last accessed October 14, 2020, https://www.mayoclinic.org/diseases-conditions/ovarian-hyperstimulation-syndrome-ohss/symptoms-causes/syc-20354697.

25 "What is Intracytoplasmic Sperm Injection (ICSI)?" American Society for Reproductive Medicine, revised 2014, https://www.reproductivefacts.org/news-and-publications/patient-fact-sheets-and-booklets/documents/fact-sheets-and-info-booklets/what-is-intracytoplasmic-sperm-injection-icsi/.

26 American Society for Reproductive Medicine, "Age and Fertility."

27 McHaney, Sarah and Jacobson, Rebecca (Inside Energy), "7 Things Every Woman Should Know Before Freezing Her Eggs," PBS News Hour, December 10, 2014, https://www.pbs.org/newshour/science/freeze-eggs#.

28 Mayo Clinic, "Ovarian Hyperstimulation Syndrome."

29 MacMillan, Carrie, "Is Egg Freezing Right for You?" Yale Medicine (blog), May 29, 2019, https://www.yalemedicine.org/stories/egg-freezing-fertility/.

30 Society for Assisted Reproductive Technology, "Fresh and Frozen Embryo Transfers."

31 "National Summary Report," Society for Assisted Reproductive Technology, 2017 data, last accessed October 14, 2020, https://www.sartcorsonline.com/rptCSR_PublicMultYear.aspx?reportingYear=2017.

32 Society for Assisted Reproductive Technology, "Fresh and Frozen Embryo Transfers."

33 Igenomix, "What to Know About Endometrial Receptivity Analysis."

34 "Infertility FAQs," Centers for Disease Control and Prevention, last accessed October 15, 2020, https://www.cdc.gov/reproductivehealth/infertility/index.htm.

35 Shirazi, Talia, "How Your Chances of Conceiving are Affected by Your Cycle, Age, Birth Control, Health Conditions (And More)," A Modern Fertility Blog, March 3, 2020, https://modernfertility.com/blog/chances-of-conception/.

36 American Society for Reproductive Medicine, "Age and Fertility."

37 "IUI Success Rates," Attain Fertility, last accessed October 15, 2020, https://attainfertility.com/understanding-fertility/treatment-options/iui/success-rates/.

38 Society for Assisted Reproductive Technology, "National Summary Report."

39 Cleveland Clinic, "Adenomyosis."

40 Centers for Disease Control and Prevention, "Infertility FAQs."

41 "Infertility Causes," Cleveland Clinic, last reviewed by a Cleveland Clinic medical professional on May 10, 2016, last accessed November 15, 2020, https://my.clevelandclinic.org/health/diseases/16083-infertility-causes.

42 Smith ADAC, Tilling K, Nelson SM, Lawlor DA, "Live-Birth Rate Associated With Repeat In Vitro Fertilization Treatment Cycles," JAMA, 314,24 (2015): 2654–2662, doi:10.1001/jama.2015.17296.

43 University of Turku, "Social laughter releases endorphins in the brain," ScienceDaily, last accessed October 16, 2020, www.sciencedaily.com/releases/2017/06/170601124121.htm.

44 "The Power of Pets: Health Benefits of Human-Animal Interactions," NIH News in Health, February 2018, https://newsinhealth.nih.gov/2018/02/power-pets.

45 "What is HCG?" American Pregnancy Association, April 25, 2019, https://americanpregnancy.org/getting-pregnant/hcg-levels-71048.

46 "Dilation and Curettage (D&C)," Mayo Clinic, October 29, 2019, https://www.mayoclinic.org/tests-procedures/dilation-and-curettage/about/pac-20384910.

47 "How Common is Miscarriage?" Tommy's, last reviewed April 10, 2018, https://www.tommys.org/pregnancy-information/im-pregnant/early-pregnancy/how-common-miscarriage.

48 "Causes of Miscarriage," Tommy's, last reviewed March 12, 2020, https://www.tommys.org/pregnancy-information/pregnancy-complications/baby-loss/miscarriage/causes-miscarriage.

49 "What Causes Depression?" Harvard Health Publishing, Harvard Medical School, published June 2009, last updated June 24, 2019, https://www.health.harvard.edu/mind-and-mood/what-causes-depression.

50 Shapiro, Connie, PhD, "New Research on Stress and Infertility," Psychology Today, August 20, 2010, https://www.psychologytoday.com/us/blog/when-youre-not-expecting/201008/new-research-stress-and-infertility#.

51 Marchant, NL, Lovland, LR, Jones, R et al., "Repetitive Negative Thinking is Associated with Amyloid, Tau, and Cognitive decline," *Alzheimer's Dement*, 16 (2020): 1054-1064, https://doi.org/10.1002/alz.12116.

52 Centers for Disease Control and Prevention, "Infertility FAQs."

53 "State Laws Related to Insurance Coverage for Infertility Treatment," National Conference of State Legislatures, June 12, 2019, https://www.ncsl.org/research/health/insurance-coverage-for-infertility-laws.aspx; Klein, Amy, "I.V.F. is Expensive. Here's How to Bring Down the Cost," *New York Times*, April 18, 2020, https://www.nytimes.com/article/ivf-treatment-costs-guide.html.

54 Smith, "Live-Birth Rate," 2654-2662.

55 Semega, Jessica et al., "Income and Poverty in the United States: 2019," United States Census Bureau, Report No. P60-270, September 15, 2020, https://www.census.gov/library/publications/2020/demo/p60-270.html.

56 "Infertility Coverage by State," Resolve, last accessed October 22, 2020, https://resolve.org/what-are-my-options/insurance-coverage/infertility-coverage-state/.

57 Vega, Tanzina, "Infertility, Endured Through a Prism of Race," *New York Times*, April 25, 2014, https://www.nytimes.

com/2014/04/26/us/infertility-endured-through-a-prism-of-race.html.

58 Tranell, Kim, "'My Final IVF Cycle Was Canceled Due To COVID-19'," *Women's Health Magazine*, March 24, 2020, https://www.womenshealthmag.com/health/a31905445/ivf-asrm-coronavirus-essay/.

59 Rooney, Kristin L, and Alice D Domar, "The Relationship Between Stress and Infertility," *Dialogues in Clinical Neuroscience*, 20, 1 (2018): 41-47, doi:10.31887/DCNS.2018.20.1/klrooney.

60 American Society for Reproductive Medicine, "What is Intracytoplasmic Sperm Injection (ICSI)?"

61 "Preimplantation Genetic Testing," American Society for Reproductive Medicine, revised 2014, https://www.reproductivefacts.org/news-and-publications/patient-fact-sheets-and-booklets/documents/fact-sheets-and-info-booklets/preimplantation-genetic-testing/.

62 "PGT-A and PGS Genetic Screening of Embryos ," FertilityIQ, last accessed October 26, 2020, https://www.fertilityiq.com/ivf-in-vitro-fertilization/pgs-genetic-screening-of-embryos#what-is-pgs-genetic-screening.

63 Cleveland Clinic, "Adenomyosis."

64 Donaldson-Evans, Catherine, "Subchorionic Bleeding During Pregnancy," What to Expect, medically reviewed by Sarah Obican, M.D. on October 8, 2020, last accessed October 26, 2020, https://www.whattoexpect.com/pregnancy/pregnancy-health/complications/subchorionic-bleeding.aspx#.

65 "WHO Director-General's opening remarks at the media briefing on COVID-19," World Health Organization, March 11, 2020, https://www.who.int/dg/speeches/detail/who-director-general-s-opening-remarks-at-the-media-briefing-on-covid-19---11-march-2020.

66 "Proclamation on Declaring a National Emergency Concerning the Novel Coronavirus Disease (COVID-19) Outbreak," The White House, March 13, 2020, https://www.whitehouse.gov/presidential-actions/

    proclamation-declaring-national-emergency-concerning-novel-coronavirus-disease-covid-19-outbreak/.

67 "Patient Management and Clinical Recommendations During the Coronavirus (COVID-19) Pandemic," American Society for Reproductive Medicine, March 17, 2020, https://www.asrm.org/globalassets/asrm/asrm-content/news-and-publications/covid-19/covidtaskforce.pdf.

68 Cleveland Clinic, "Adenomyosis."

69 Cleveland Clinic, "Endometriosis."

70 Mayo Clinic, "Polycystic Ovary Syndrome (PCOS)."

71 American Society for Reproductive Medicine, "Ovarian Reserve."

72 American Society for Reproductive Medicine, "Ovarian Reserve."

73 American Society for Reproductive Medicine, "Ovarian Reserve."

74 "Progesterone and Pregnancy: A Vital Connection," Resolve, last accessed October 8, 2020, https://resolve.org/infertility-101/the-female-body/progesterone-pregnancy-vital-connection/.

75 "Thyroid Function Tests," American Thyroid Association, last accessed October 8, 2020, https://www.thyroid.org/thyroid-function-tests/.

76 Tobah, "Hypothyroidism and Infertility: Any Connection?"

77 The American College of Obstetricians and Gynecologists, "Carrier Screening."

78 American Society for Reproductive Medicine, "Preimplantation Genetic Testing."

79 Johns Hopkins Medicine, "Pelvic Ultrasound."

80 American Society for Reproductive Medicine, "Saline Infusion Sonohysterogram (SHG)."

81 American Society for Reproductive Medicine, "Hysterosalpingogram (HSG)."

82 American Society for Reproductive Medicine, "Laparoscopy and Hysteroscopy."

83 Igenomix, "What to Know About Endometrial Receptivity Analysis."

84 Fertility Center of Illinois, "Everything You Need to Know About Timed Intercourse."

85 Resolve, "What is IUI?"

86 Resolve, "What is IVF?"

87 Society for Assisted Reproductive Technology, "Fresh and Frozen Embryo Transfers."

88 American Society for Reproductive Medicine, "What is Intracytoplasmic Sperm Injection (ICSI)?"

89 "Miscarriage," Planned Parenthood, last accessed October 8, 2020, https://www.plannedparenthood.org/learn/pregnancy/miscarriage.

90 "What is Stillbirth?" Centers for Disease Control and Prevention, last accessed October 8, 2020, https://www.cdc.gov/ncbddd/stillbirth/facts.html.

91 Centers for Disease Control and Prevention, "What is Stillbirth?"

ACKNOWLEDGEMENTS

I self-publish my books under my own publishing company, Mortal Ink Press, LLC. For most of my books, I hire out a good amount of the work I need to do, such as cover design and proofreading. In this case, the project felt extremely personal. So I designed the cover for this book and did the typesetting, formatting, and editing myself. That's why the endnotes are so impressive. Obviously. This is entirely my story in my voice and my voice alone.

Thanks to my husband Malcolm for enthusiastically supporting this project, listening to every chapter, writing the foreword, and letting me share all our infertility laundry with the world. You are an amazing partner. There is no one else I can imagine going through this journey with.

Thanks also to our doctors, who have provided us with excellent medical treatment over the years. I do not expect any of you to be gods, so if you happen to read this and you feel you were portrayed in some negative light, know that I never intended that. Not everything that has ever happened to me at a fertility clinic has been perfectly ideal, but that is not inconsistent with my belief that I've had great doctors.

ABOUT THE AUTHOR

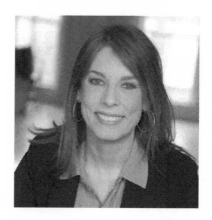

Sandra L. Vasher is an indie writer and publisher, recovering lawyer, dreamer, consultant, blogger, serial entrepreneur, and mommy of a brand new baby and a very spoiled dog. (Oooh, see how I sneaked that unambiguous end in later for you here?) She enjoys long drives in fall weather, do-it-yourself projects, animated movies and cartoons, fanfiction, red wine, traveling everywhere, and baking sweet and savory treats.

Before the pandemic, she could often be found trying not to hunch over her computer at her favorite coffee shops in Raleigh, North Carolina. Now, you can find her writing virtually on the WordStitch channel at https://www.youtube.com/c/WordStitchWriteIns. You can also follow Sandy online at sandyvasher.com.

OTHER BOOKS
By Sandra L. Vasher

MORTAL HERITANCE

Sisters of the Perilous Heart
Kingdoms of the Frozen Dead (January 2021)

THE IMMORTAL MISTAKES

Stella Rose Gold for Eternity
Lizzy Dupree and the Thousand-Year Crush
Mila Hildebrand is Forever Not Yours

3 SIMPLE STEPS TO
HELP AN INDIE

This book was independently published by a writer, not a traditional publishing house. But indie writing is more than a DIY hobby; it's a full-time business. The indie writer of this book needs your support to make that business successful. Here's what you can do to make sure you get a sequel:

 ## REVIEW THE BOOK

 Write a short, honest review and post it online. You can usually review wherever you bought the book and on Goodreads.

 ## RECOMMEND THE BOOK TO A FRIEND

If you liked the book, tell someone about it! This is how most readers decide what to read next.

 ## SUBSCRIBE

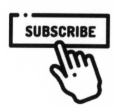 Go to the writer's website and click "subscribe." This will put you on the writer's list of readers to reach out to about news, events, giveaways, and opportunities to be part of the launch team for her next book. This writer's website is:

https://sandyvasher.com

THANK YOU!

Made in the USA
Middletown, DE
04 December 2021

54249660R00203